Neonatal and Pediatric Critical Care Plans

D1527034

NURSING DIAGNOSIS
POCKET GUIDE

Neonatal and Pediatric Critical Care Plans

SHARON ENNIS AXTON, RN, PNP, MS
Nursing Specialist in Pediatric Pulmonary Nursing
Associate Professor of Clinical Nursing
Texas Tech University
Health Sciences Center, School of Nursing
Lubbock, Texas

TERRY FUGATE, RN, BSN
formerly Adjunct/Associate Faculty
Texas Tech University
Health Sciences Center, School of Nursing
Lubbock, Texas

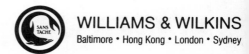

WILLIAMS & WILKINS
Baltimore • Hong Kong • London • Sydney

Editor: Susan M. Glover
Associate Editor: Marjorie Kidd Keating
Copy Editor: Linda Forlifer
Design: Bob Och
Production: Charles E. Zeller

Copyright © 1989
Williams & Wilkins
428 East Preston Street
Baltimore, MD 21202, U.S.A.

All rights reserved. This book is protected by copyright. No part of this book may be reproduced in any form or by any means, including photocopying, or utilized by any information storage and retrieval system without written permission from the copyright owner.

Accurate indications, adverse reactions, and dosage schedules for drugs are provided in this book, but it is possible that they may change. The reader is urged to review the package information data of the manufacturers of the medications mentioned.

Printed in the United States of America

Library of Congress Cataloging in Publication Data

Main entry under title:

Axton, Sharon Ennis.
  Neonatal and pediatric critical care plans / Sharon Ennis Axton.
  Terry Fugate.
      p.   cm. — (Nursing diagnosis pocket guide)

     Includes index.
     ISBN 0-683-00299-6
     1. Neonatal intensive care. 2. Pediatric intensive care.
3. Nursing care plans. I. Fugate, Terry II. Title.
III. Series.
    [DNLM: 1. Critical Care—in infancy & childhood—handbooks.
2. Neonatology—handbooks. 3. Neonatology—nurses' instruction.
4. Nursing Process—methods—handbooks. 5. Pediatric Nursing—
methods—handbooks. WY 39 A972na]
RJ253.5.A97 1989   618.92'0028—dc19
DNLM/DLC   88-27643
for Library of Congress   CIP

89 90 91 92 93
1 2 3 4 5 6 7 8 9 10

Foreword

In times of insufficient staffing, nurses emphasize time management strategies. In times of sufficient staffing, nurses emphasize comprehensive care strategies. These strategies are not exclusive; rather they complement each other. This book integrates a time-effective approach with comprehensive care.

In acute care situations, patients have clearly established medical diagnoses. Therefore, being able to relate nursing diagnoses, goals, and measures to medical diagnoses in an efficient manner is valuable to the professional nurse. Again, this book provides an interrelationship of the nursing framework with the medical approach.

With numerous nursing texts focusing on critical care related to children and neonates, why would a professional nurse choose this text as an essential reference? Several reasons come to mind—readability, quick reference format, and practice-based content.

The guiding principle of the Texas Tech University Health Sciences Center School of Nursing is reintegration, meaning a return to the multiple-focus role of nurses. This principle is demonstrated through the use of unique nursing talents in the areas of education, clinical practice, scholarly activity, and service to the institution and the community. The motivation for this book was Sharon Axton's realization that there were problems with using nursing care plans, diagnoses, and consistent approaches to care in the clinical arena. It was necessary for the undergraduate curriculum to address these problems. In preparing this book, Sharon Axton has "pulled together" what she teaches and what happens in the real world of practice. As she uses the information in external workshops and conferences, she will provide service to the community. She has demonstrated the reintegrated role and simultaneously has served as a mentor to Terry Fugate.

During the past few years, I have observed students rapidly incorporate into their practice the kind of information that Sharon Axton and Terry Fugate have generated. I have heard comments from people external to our school of nursing referring to *Neonatal and Pediatric Care Plans*, Sharon Axton's first text. This present book represents the culmination of a major collaborative effort of two professional nurses to benefit all who provide care to children and neonates in critical care settings. I hope that the real impact of this book is demonstrated in the enhanced nursing care that clients receive.

Pat S. Yoder Wise, RN, EdD
Editor
The Journal of Continuing Education in Nursing
Executive Associate Dean and Professor
Texas Tech University Health Sciences Center
School of Nursing
Lubbock, Texas

Preface   The desire to write a book of nursing care plans for critically ill neonates and children arose from our past experience as practicing nurses and educators. We realized that a source was needed to help identify nursing diagnoses for these patients and their families. This need was verified by both nursing students and nurses practicing in these areas.

Pediatric critical care nurses and neonatal nurses are ever present at the patient's bedside, constantly assessing, planning, implementing, and evaluating the care needed by the patient and the family. From our past experience and observation of other nurses in these settings, it has become evident that time management is often a major concern. Our hope is that this book will allow the formation of quick and accurate nursing diagnoses and will provide the basis for the development of individualized nursing care plans. To facilitate this process, we decided to correlate several nursing diagnoses with some of the most common medical diagnoses found in pediatric critical care units and neonatal units.

Most of the nursing diagnoses are those accepted and published by the North American Nursing Diagnosis Association (NANDA). On a few occasions, it was necessary to utilize some diagnoses that have not yet been approved.

We would like to express our appreciation to all of our colleagues (educators and practicing nurses) who, through their encouragement and support, have contributed to our personal and professional growth. We would also like to acknowledge our nursing students for their enthusiasm, which is a continual source of inspiration.

Sharon Ennis Axton
Terry Fugate

Contents

Introduction The goal of *Neonatal and Pediatric Critical Care Plans* is to assist practicing nurses, nurse educators, and students in implementing the nursing process for critically ill neonatal and pediatric patients. This book provides a quick reference for correlating frequently encountered neonatal and pediatric medical diagnoses with nursing diagnoses.

Each diagnostic entry has a standard set of components:

Medical Diagnosis

Pathophysiology: This is a basic and brief overview of the pathophysiology of the medical diagnosis.

Primary Nursing Diagnosis: This can be stated as either actual or potential. The nurse writing the care plan makes this determination.

Definition: This refers only to the nursing diagnosis and not to the medical diagnosis.

Possibly Related to: The rationale for the selection of each nursing diagnosis is inherent in this statement.

Characteristics: These are of the selected primary nursing diagnosis and of the identified medical diagnosis. The list presents possible signs and symptoms of the identified medical diagnosis.

Expected Outcomes: Listing expected outcomes is the next step in the nursing process after identification of the nursing diagnosis. Expected outcomes may be listed on a nursing care plan as pa-

tient goals or objectives. Outcomes are written as specifically as possible so they are measurable and can be easily evaluated. Directions are sometimes included to help individualize the expected outcomes for each infant/child. For example, in the pediatric section, an expected outcome might read as follows:

Child will have adequate cardiac output as evidenced by
  a. heart rate within acceptable range (state specific highest and lowest rates for each child)

To individualize this statement, the nurse needs to include the highest and lowest acceptable heart rates for each child. The range will vary depending upon age and disease state. The expected outcome for a 1-month-old infant with normal cardiac function would read:

Child will have adequate cardiac output as evidenced by
  a. heart rate of 100 to 160 beats/ minute

Possible Nursing Interventions: These are ways in which the nurse can assist the infant/child and/or family to achieve the expected outcomes. Some of these interventions are *independent* nursing actions, whereas others are *collaborative* (as the nurse implements the physician's orders). For example, a nursing intervention to "elevate the head of the bed at a 30° angle" could be instituted for an infant/child with increased intracranial pressure without a specific order from the physician. This would be

an independent nursing intervention. A nursing intervention to "ensure that antibiotic is administered on schedule" is dependent upon the physician's order.

Evaluation for Charting: This is the final step in the nursing process. This section evaluates the expected outcomes and, to some extent, the identified nursing interventions. Statements made here direct the reader to describe or state results. For example, the reader may be directed to "describe breath sounds." This would be correlated with the expected outcome, "infant/child will have clear and equal breath sounds," and with a nursing intervention such as "assess and record infant/child's breath sounds every 2 hours and PRN."

The evaluation statement may need to be changed frequently. For this reason the nurse may wish to include this part of the nursing process in the daily charting; if so, the nurse would note on the nursing care plan under the evaluation column, "See nurses' notes," and state date, time, and initials.

Associated Nursing Diagnoses: Following the primary nursing diagnosis are one to three nursing diagnoses (actual or potential) that are prioritized and carried through the nursing process.

Related Nursing Diagnoses: These are nursing diagnoses that are most likely to be included in a nursing care plan for an infant/child with the stated medical diagnosis. Many of these nursing diagnoses are either potential or actual nursing diagnoses; the nurse determines which.

The related nursing diagnoses are in priority order for an infant/child with the stated medical diagnosis. However, the needs and condition of the infant/child will determine whether the nurse must reorder the priorities. All related nursing diagnoses are completely developed through the nursing process and can be found in the text; refer to the index for location.

A separate section is included on those nursing diagnoses that are unrelated to specific medical diagnoses. All such diagnoses have been included in the *Related Nursing Diagnoses*.

To use this book most efficiently, scan the Contents for the applicable medical diagnosis. After finding it in the text, review the accompanying nursing care plan and related nursing diagnoses, and select the appropriate expected outcomes and nursing interventions. Write those on the nursing care plan and then implement them. Later, at intervals that you designate when writing the care plan, evaluate the infant/child's response to your nursing interventions and record your findings.

With this Nursing Diagnosis Pocket Guide, *Neonatal and Pediatric Critical Care Plans*, you will organize your nursing practice around nursing diagnoses, the professional level of practice.

Section 1
Neonatal Critical Care Plans

Medical Diagnosis

INTRAVENTRICULAR HEMORRHAGE

Pathophysiology

Intraventricular hemorrhage (IVH) is bleeding from the cerebral capillaries that can extend into the ventricles. The bleeding occurs in the subependymal germinal matrix, which is an area (present only in infants born before 40 weeks gestation) located next to the ventricles. This matrix provides only minimal support for the blood vessels running through it. The tiny, fragile capillaries in the germinal matrix can be ruptured easily by hypoxic-ischemic events. Obstruction of cerebral flow and hydrocephalus can result.

The incidence of IVH is greater than 50% in infants born before 30 weeks gestation and weighing less than 1250 grams. An IVH is usually graded I through IV. Grade I is the mildest and most common form. The blood is restricted to the area of the germinal matrix and does not enter the ventricles. This type of hemorrhage usually resolves without abnormalities. Grade IV, the most serious, includes bleeding into the ventricles and the surrounding brain tissue.

Primary Nursing Diagnosis

ALTERATION IN LEVEL OF CONSCIOUSNESS

Definition

Reduced or impaired state of awareness: can range from mild to complete impairment

Possibly Related to

- Hypoxic-ischemic events

- Cerebral trauma and depression of cerebral blood flow secondary to vaginal delivery
- Venous congestion or increased cerebral venous pressure
- Arterial overperfusion
- Impaired autoregulation of the cerebral circulation
- Complication from use of volume expanders
- Increased intrapleural pressure
- Complication of a pneumothorax (from transmission of the positive pressure from the ventilator in the pleural space)
- Complication from use of hyperosmolar solutions (bicarbonate)

Characteristics

Initial Signs

Subtle changes in tone or activity

Brief multifocal seizures

Minor alterations in consciousness

Transient apnea

Bradycardia

Mild hypotension

Full anterior fontanel

A fall in hematrocrit or failure of hematocrit to rise with blood transfusion

Unexplained fluctuations in temperature

Unexplained jaundice

Sudden appearance of hyperglycemia or hypoglycemia

Late Signs

Ashen color

Unresponsiveness

Abrupt decrease in muscular and spontaneous activity

Focal or major motor seizures and abnormal eye movements

Worsening respiratory status despite previously adequate ventilatory support

Severe hypotension

Bulging fontanel, split sutures

Increased head circumference

Shock

Expected Outcomes

Infant will maintain an appropriate level of consciousness as evidenced by

a. adequate tone
b. spontaneous and equal movement of all extremities
c. absence of seizure activity
d. lack of apnea and ashen color
e. heart rate within acceptable range of 100 to 160 beats/minute
f. B/P within acceptable range of 64/30 to 96/62 mm Hg
g. flat fontanel
h. hematocrit within acceptable range of 44 to 72%
i. temperature within acceptable range of 36.5° to 37.2° C
j. absence of jaundice
k. serum glucose within acceptable range of 25 to 60 mg/dl
l. stable ventilator settings
m. stable head circumference

Possible Nursing Interventions

• Assess and record the following every 2 hours and PRN

—neurologic signs
—anterior fontanel condition
—vital signs
—signs/symptoms of alteration in level of consciousness (such as those listed under "Characteristics")

- Keep accurate record of intake and output. Avoid rapid IV infusion or rapid IV pushes.
- Measure and record head circumference daily.
- Reduce excessive stressors such as excessive handling, bright lights, and noise.
- Organize nursing care to minimize disturbing and stimulating the infant.
- Elevate head of bed at a 30° angle. Position head in midline.

Evaluation for Charting

- Describe neurologic signs.
- State range of vital signs.
- Describe condition of anterior fontanel.
- Describe any signs/symptoms of alteration in level of consciousness (such as those listed under "Characteristics").
- State head circumference and determine whether it is an increase or decrease from the previous measurement.
- State intake and output.
- Describe any therapeutic measures used to decrease intracranial pressure and their effectiveness.
- Note whether head of bed was maintained at a 30° angle and whether head was kept in a midline position.

Nursing Diagnosis

IMPAIRED GAS EXCHANGE

Definition

Alteration in the exchange of oxygen and carbon dioxide in the lungs and/or at the cellular level

Possibly Related to

- Increased intrapleural pressure
- Gestational age
- Immature lung tissue

Characteristics
Apnea
Hypercapnia
Hypoxemia
Worsening respiratory status despite previously adequate ventilatory support

Expected Outcomes
Infant will maintain adequate gas exchange as evidenced by

    a. respiratory rate within acceptable range of 30 to 60 breaths/minute
    b. arterial blood gas values within acceptable range (state specific highest and lowest values for each infant)
    c. stable ventilator settings

Possible Nursing Interventions
- Assess and record

    —respiratory rate every 2 hours and PRN
    —arterial blood gas values when indicated. Notify physician if results are out of the stated range.
    —any signs/symptoms of impaired gas exchange (such as those listed under "Characteristics") every 2 hours and PRN

- Ensure that oxygen is being delivered in the correct amount and by the correct route. Record percentage of liter flow and route of delivery. Assess and record effectiveness of treatment.
- Assess patency of endotracheal tube by listening to breath sounds frequently (every 30 minutes to 1 hour).
- Avoid interrupting ventilation as much as possible and minimize frequency of suctioning if possible. Use sterile technique when suctioning

and record amount and characteristics of secretions.
- Check ventilator settings (FiO2, Rate, PIP or TV, PEEP/CPAP) every 15 minutes. Record every 1 to 2 hours.

Evaluation for Charting

- State highest and lowest respiratory rate.
- State highest and lowest arterial blood gas values and state the on-going physiologic process (i.e., respiratory acidosis).
- Describe any signs/symptoms of impaired gas exchange noted (such as those listed under "Characteristics").
- State type of endotracheal tube in place and ventilator settings.
- Describe frequency, amount, and characteristics of secretions.

Related Nursing Diagnoses

ALTERATION IN COMFORT related to increased intracranial pressure

DECREASED CARDIAC OUTPUT related to
   a. hypoxia
   b. venous congestion
   c. arterial overperfusion

INEFFECTIVE FAMILY COPING related to
   a. possibility of neurologically handicapped infant
   b. increased length of hospital stay

DEVELOPMENTAL DELAY related to increased intracranial pressure

Medical Diagnosis	# BRONCHOPULMONARY DYSPLASIA
Pathophysiology	Bronchopulmonary dysplasia (BPD) is a progressive generalized lung disease that results in thickening and necrosis of the alveolar walls and the basement membranes. It is characterized by atelectasis and fibrosis. It results from prolonged oxygen therapy and ventilatory assistance. Prevention of BPD is not always possible. Attempts should be made to keep inspired oxygen tensions as low as possible while maintaining adequate arterial oxygen tension. Ventilator pressures should be reduced when possible to prevent barotrauma.
Primary Nursing Diagnosis	## IMPAIRED GAS EXCHANGE
Definition	Alteration in the exchange of oxygen and carbon dioxide in the lungs and/or at the cellular level
Possibly Related to	<ul><li>Long-term ventilator therapy</li><li>Barotrauma from mechanical ventilation</li><li>High oxygen concentration</li><li>Alveolar rupture or pulmonary interstitial emphysema</li></ul>
Characteristics	Tachypnea Retractions Nasal flaring Rales Diminished or unequal breath sounds Deterioration of arterial blood gas values Cyanosis Chest x-ray film ultimately reveals opacification, cystic infiltrates, and increased density

**Expected
Outcomes** Infant will maintain adequate gas exchange as evidenced by

a. respiratory rate within acceptable range of 30 to 60 breaths/minute
b. clear and equal breath sounds
c. lack of

—retractions
—nasal flaring
—cyanosis

d. arterial blood gas values within acceptable range (state specific highest and lowest values for each infant)
e. clear chest x-ray

**Possible Nursing
Interventions** • Assess and record

—respiratory rate and breath sounds every 2 hours and PRN
—signs/symptoms of impaired gas exchange (such as those listed under "Characteristics") every 2 hours and PRN
—arterial blood gas values when indicated. Notify physician if results are out of the stated range.

• Ensure that oxygen is being delivered in the correct amount and route. Record percentage of liter flow and route of delivery. Assess and record effectiveness of treatment.
• Assess patency of endotracheal tube by listening to breath sounds frequently (every 30 minutes to 1 hour).
• Suction endotracheal tube using sterile technique every 2 to 3 hours and PRN. Record amount and characteristics of secretions.

- Check ventilator settings (FiO2, Rate, PIP or TV, PEEP/CPAP) every 15 minutes. Record every 1 to 2 hours.
- Ensure that chest physiotherapy is being done effectively and gently on schedule.
- Check and record results of chest x-ray when indicated.
- Change infant's position every 2 hours.

Evaluation for Charting

- State highest and lowest respiratory rates.
- Describe breath sounds.
- State highest and lowest arterial blood gas values and state the on-going physiologic process (i.e., respiratory acidosis).
- Describe any signs/symptoms of impaired gas exchange noted (such as those listed under "Characteristics").
- State amount, route, and effectiveness of oxygen therapy.
- Describe amount and characteristics of secretions.
- State ventilator settings.
- State whether the chest physiotherapy treatments were effective in improving gas exchange.
- Describe results of chest x-ray if available.
- State whether infant's position was changed every 2 hours.

Nursing Diagnosis   **DECREASED CARDIAC OUTPUT**

Definition   A decrease in the amount of blood that leaves the left ventricle

Possibly Related to   Increased pulmonary vascular resistance

Characteristics	Tachycardia
	Tachypnea
	Dyspnea
	Cyanosis
	Feeding difficulties
	Fatigue

Expected Outcomes

Infant will maintain an adequate cardiac output as evidenced by

   a. heart rate within acceptable range of 100 to 160 beats/minute
   b. respiratory rate within acceptable range of 30 to 60 breaths/minute
   c. strong and equal pulses bilaterally
   d. lack of

      —cyanosis
      —fatigue
      —feeding difficulties

Possible Nursing Interventions

• Assess and record every 2 hours and PRN

   —heart and respiratory rates
   —breath sounds
   —femoral, brachial, and pedal pulses
   —any signs/symptoms of decreased cardiac output (such as those listed under "Characteristics")

• Organize nursing care to allow rest periods to decrease workload on the heart.
• Elevate head of bed at a 30° angle.

Evaluation for Charting

• State highest lowest heart and respiratory rates.
• Describe breath sounds.
• State presence and strength of peripheral pulses.
• Describe any signs/symptoms of decreased cardiac output (such as those listed under "Characteristics").

Related Nursing Diagnoses

- Note whether infant was elevated at a 30° angle.

POTENTIAL FOR INFECTION related to increased pulmonary secretions

ALTERATION IN LEVEL OF CONSCIOUSNESS related to decreased oxygenation

INEFFECTIVE FAMILY COPING related to long-term hospitalization of infant

ALTERATION IN NUTRITION: LESS THAN BODY REQUIREMENTS related to respiratory distress

| Medical Diagnosis | # CONGENITAL DIAPHRAGMATIC HERNIA |

Medical Diagnosis

CONGENITAL DIAPHRAGMATIC HERNIA

Pathophysiology

A congenital defect of the diaphragm that allows abdominal contents (stomach, large part of the intestines, and sometimes the spleen and liver) to extend into the thoracic cavity. The defect results from failure of the pleuroperitoneal canal to close completely during fetal development. It usually occurs in full-term infants, is more common on the left (85%) than on the right side, and can be bilateral (1 to 2%). Cardiac output and pulmonary gas exchange is compromised as a result of the abdominal contents displacing the heart and lungs. The lung on the affected side is often underdeveloped (hypoplastic).

Primary Nursing Diagnosis

IMPAIRED GAS EXCHANGE

Definition

Alteration in the exchange of oxygen and carbon dioxide in the lungs and/or at the cellular level

Possibly Related to

Inability of the lung to expand secondary to protrusion of the abdominal contents into the thoracic cavity

Characteristics

Cyanosis

Dyspnea

Hypoxemia

Tachypnea

Severe acidosis

Diminished breath sounds in the involved hemithorax

Audible bowel sounds in the thoracic cavity

X-ray revealing gas-filled intestinal loops in the chest

Scaphoid abdomen (sometimes)

**Expected
Outcomes**   Infant will maintain adequate gas exchange (until emergency surgery can be
arranged) as evidenced by

  a. lack of

    —extreme cyanosis
    —dyspnea

  b. clear breath sounds on unaffected
     side of chest
  c. arterial blood gas values within ac-
     ceptable range (state specific
     highest and lowest values for each
     infant)
  d. respiratory rate within acceptable
     range of 30 to 60 breaths/minute

**Possible Nursing
Interventions**   • Assess and record

    —respiratory rate every 2 hours and
     PRN
    —breath sounds every 2 hours and
     PRN
    —signs/symptoms of impaired gas
     exchange (such as those listed
     under "Characteristics") every 2
     hours and PRN
    —arterial blood gas values when in-
     dicated

  • Ensure that oxygen is being deliv-
    ered in the correct amount and by
    the correct route. Record percentage
    of liter flow and route of delivery.
    State effectiveness of treatment.
  • Assess patency of endotracheal tube
    by listening to breath sounds fre-
    quently (every 30 minutes to 1 hour).
  • Suction endotracheal tube using ster-
    ile technique every 2 to 3 hours and
    PRN. Record characteristics of secre-
    tions.

- Check ventilator settings (FiO2, Rate, PIP or TV) every 15 minutes. Record every 1 to 2 hours. Low ventilatory pressures without PEEP/CPAP and rapid rates are generally used to ventilate patient. There is an increased chance of a pneumothorax when positive pressure is used due to the uneven distribution of pressure (most of the pressure goes to the unaffected side).
- Position infant with the head and thorax higher than the abdomen to help encourage downward displacement of the abdominal contents.
- Prevent infant from crying whenever possible by utilizing comfort measures and organizing care so that distressing procedures can be done at one time. Crying will allow the infant to swallow air, which will result in increased respiratory distress.
- Ensure that a nasogastric tube is placed correctly and connected to suction in order to decompress the stomach.
- Ensure that antibiotics are administered on schedule. Assess and record any side effects (such as diarrhea or rash).
- Check and record results of chest x-ray if available.

Evaluation for Charting

- Describe breath sounds and any signs/symptoms of impaired gas exchange (such as those listed under "Characteristics").
- State highest and lowest respiratory rates.
- State highest and lowest arterial blood gas values and state the on-go-

ing physiologic process (i.e., respiratory acidosis).
- State amount, route, and effectiveness of oxygen therapy.
- State type of endotracheal tube and ventilator settings.
- Describe amount and characteristics of secretions.
- State whether infant was maintained in a head-elevated position.
- Describe any successful measures used to decrease crying.
- State whether nasogastric suctioning was effective in reducing abdominal distention.
- State whether antibiotics were administered on schedule. Describe any side effects.
- State results of chest x-ray if available.

Nursing Diagnosis

DECREASED CARDIAC OUTPUT

Definition

A decrease in the amount of blood that leaves the left ventricle

Possibly Related to

Mediastinal shift secondary to protrusion of abdominal contents into the thoracic cavity

Characteristics

Heart sounds shifted to one side

X-ray revealing heart displaced to one side of chest

Cyanosis

Dyspnea

Expected Outcomes

Infant will maintain adequate cardiac output as evidenced by

    a. heart rate within acceptable range of 100 to 160 beats/minute

    b. lack of

      —severe cyanosis

      —dyspnea

**Possible Nursing
Interventions**

—increasing displacement of heart to one side of chest

- Assess and record every 2 hours and PRN

    —heart sounds and rate
    —signs/symptoms of decreased cardiac output (such as those listed under "Characteristics")

- Check and record results of chest x-ray if available.
- Organize nursing care so infant will have only minimal stimulation (and decreased crying) to improve oxygenation and decrease workload on the heart.
- Keep accurate intake and output. Infant will be NPO and will receive IV fluids probably through a UAC. Fluid overload could decrease cardiac output.

**Evaluation
for Charting**

- Describe heart sounds and their position.
- State highest and lowest heart rates.
- Describe any signs/symptoms of decreased cardiac output (such as those listed under "Characteristics").
- State results of chest x-ray if available.
- State whether infant was only minimally stimulated and whether this helped to improve oxygenation and cardiac output.
- State intake and output.

**Related Nursing
Diagnoses**

POTENTIAL FOR INFECTION related to emergency surgery and invasive procedures

INEFFECTIVE FAMILY COPING related to

    a. emergency surgical procedure required for newborn

    b. high fatality rate of illness

PARENTAL KNOWLEDGE DEFICIT related to

    a. emergency surgery

    b. new treatments such as ECMO (extracorporeal membrane oxygenation) and/or high frequency ventilation

ALTERATION IN NUTRITION: LESS THAN BODY REQUIREMENTS related to decreased oxygenation and displaced intestines

Medical Diagnosis

HYALINE MEMBRANE DISEASE

Pathophysiology

When an infant is born before 35 weeks gestation, hyaline membrane disease (HMD) can occur because of incomplete pulmonary maturation. The principal factor that leads to the formation of the hyaline membrane is believed to be a deceased production of surfactant. Decreased surfactant results in atelectasis, hypoxia, respiratory acidosis, and increased pulmonary vascular resistance. Hypoxia damages the capillary endothelium. The increased pulmonary vascular resistance leads to persistence of the fetal state, which causes increased blood pressure in the pulmonary circuit. The high pulmonary pressure helps to promote transudation of fluid into the alveoli. A matrix formed by fibrin entraps particles that are forced out of the vascular system, such as necrotic alveolar epithelium, red cells, and serum protein. All of these particles then join together to form the hyaline membrane. It will take several hours of breathing for the membrane to form. Infants who die during the first few hours after birth usually do not have the membrane.

Primary Nursing Diagnosis

IMPAIRED GAS EXCHANGE

Definition

Alteration in the exchange of oxygen and carbon dioxide in the lungs and/or at the cellular level

Possibly Related to

- Decreased production of surfactant
- Immature lung tissue

Characteristics

Tachypnea

Diminished or unequal breath sounds
Retractions (supracostal, intercostal, or subcostal)
Nasal flaring
Grunting
Cyanosis
Tachycardia
Abnormal blood gas values
Chest x-ray revealing a ground-glass appearance with air bronchograms

Expected Outcomes

Infant will maintain adequate gas exchange as evidenced by

a. respiratory rate within acceptable range of 30 to 60 breaths/minute
b. clear and equal breath sounds
c. mild to no retractions
d. lack of

—nasal flaring
—expiratory grunt
—cyanosis

e. heart rate within acceptable range of 100 to 160 beats/minute
f. arterial blood gas values within acceptable range (state specific highest and lowest values for each infant)
g. clear chest x-ray

Possible Nursing Interventions

- Assess and record every 2 hours and PRN

    —respiratory rate, heart rate, and breath sounds
    —signs/symptoms of impaired gas exchange (such as those listed under "Characteristics")

- Administer oxygen in correct amount and by correct route of delivery. State effectiveness of treatment.

- Assess patency of endotracheal tube by listening to breath sounds frequently (every 30 minutes to 1 hour).
- Suction endotracheal tube using sterile technique every 2 to 3 hours and PRN. Record characteristics of secretions.
- Oxygenate infant before treatments (such as suctioning) as indicated.
- Assess and record arterial blood gas results. Notify physician if results are out of the acceptable stated range.
- Check ventilator settings (FiO_2, Rate, PIP or TV, PEEP/CPAP) every 15 minutes. Record every 1 to 2 hours.
- Change infant position every 2 hours.
- Ensure that chest physiotherapy is being done effectively and gently on schedule.
- Check and record results of chest x-ray when indicated.

Evaluation for Charting

- Describe breath sounds.
- State highest and lowest respiratory and heart rates.
- Describe any signs/symptoms of impaired gas exchange (such as those listed under "Characteristics").
- State amount, route, and effectiveness of oxygen therapy.
- Describe amount and characteristics of secretions.
- State whether oxygenation before treatment was effective in reducing hypoxia.
- State highest and lowest arterial blood gas values and state the on-going physiologic process (i.e., respiratory acidosis).
- State ventilator settings.

- State whether infant's position was changed every 2 hours.
- State whether the chest physiotherapy treatments were effective in improving gas exchange.
- Describe the results of chest x-ray if available.

Nursing Diagnosis

POTENTIAL FOR INFECTION

Definition

A condition in which the body is invaded by microorganisms

Possibly Related to

- Invasive procedures
- Immature immune system

Characteristics

Temperature instability
Tachypnea
Apnea
Tachycardia
Lethargy

Expected Outcomes

Infant will be free of infection as evidenced by

  a. temperature between 36.5° and 37.2° C
  b. respiratory rate within acceptable range of 30 to 60 breaths/minute
  c. lack of apnea
  d. heart rate within acceptable range of 100 to 160 beats/minute
  e. lack of lethargy
  f. white blood cell count within normal limits of 9,000 to 30,000 mm^3

Possible Nursing Interventions

- Assess and record every 2 hours and PRN

  —vital signs
  —signs/symptoms of infections (such as those listed under "Characteristics")

- Maintain a neutral thermal environment.
- Ensure that antibiotics are given on schedule. Assess and record any side effects (such as rash or diarrhea).
- Assess IV site every hour for signs/ symptoms of infection or infiltration. Record findings at least once/shift.
- Use sterile technique when doing procedures such as suctioning and changing IV tubing.
- Maintain good handwashing technique, especially between patients.
- Assess parents'/visitors' knowledge of handwashing technique; correct as needed.

Evaluation for Charting

- State highest and lowest body temperatures and respiratory and heart rates.
- Describe any signs/symptoms of infection (such as those listed under "Characteristics").
- State whether a neutral thermal environment was maintained.
- State whether antibiotics were administered on schedule? Describe any side effects.
- Describe IV site.
- State whether parents/visitors demonstrated correct handwashing technique.
- State results of CBC if available.

Nursing Diagnosis

DECREASED CARDIAC OUTPUT

Definition

A decrease in the amount of blood that leaves the left ventricle

Possibly Related to Characteristics

Impaired oxygenation
Tachycardia
Tachypnea

Dyspnea
Cyanosis
Feeding difficulties
Fatigue
Edema

Expected Outcomes

Infant will maintain an adequate cardiac output as evidenced by

a. heart rate within acceptable range of 100 to 160 beats/minute
b. respiratory rate within acceptable range of 30 to 60 breaths/minute
c. strong and equal pulses bilaterally
d. lack of

   —cyanosis
   —fatigue
   —feeding difficulties
   —edema

Possible Nursing Interventions

• Assess and record every 2 hours and PRN

   —heart and respiratory rates
   —breath sounds
   —femoral, brachial, and pedal pulses
   —any signs/symptoms of decreased cardiac output (such as those listed under "Characteristics").

• Organize nursing care to allow rest periods to decrease workload on the heart.
• Elevate head of bed at a 30° angle.

Evaluation for Charting

• State highest and lowest heart and respiratory rates.
• Describe heart and breath sounds.
• State presence and strength of peripheral pulses.
• Describe any signs/symptoms of decreased cardiac output (such as those listed under "Characteristics").

- State whether infant was elevated at a 30° angle.

Nursing Diagnosis **FLUID VOLUME DEFICIT**

Definition A decrease in the amount of circulating fluid volume

Possibly Related to
- Insensible water loss from rapid respirations
- Inability to tolerate fluids by mouth

Characteristics Weight loss
Sunken fontanel
Sunken eyes
Poor skin turgor
Decreased urinary output

Expected Outcomes Infant will regain adequate fluid volume level as evidenced by

a. adequate amount of IV and/or oral fluid intake (state exact amount of intake needed for each infant)
b. weight gain of 10 to 20 grams/day
c. flat fontanel
d. lack of sunken eyes
e. rapid skin recoil
f. adequate urinary output (state acceptable minimal urinary output—0.5 to 1 ml/kg/hour)
g. urine specific gravity between 1.008 and 1.020

Possible Nursing Interventions
- Keep accurate record of intake and output.
- Weigh diapers for urine output.
- Assess and record

  —IV fluids and condition of IV site every hour

  —signs/symptoms of fluid volume deficit (such as those listed under "Characteristics") every 2 to 4 hours and PRN.

- Weigh infant daily on same scale at same time of day without clothes.
- Check and record urine specific gravity every void or as directed.

Evaluation for Charting

- State intake and output.
- State weight and determine whether it is an increase or decrease from the previous weight.
- Describe status of fontanel, eyes, and skin turgor.
- State highest and lowest urine specific gravity.

Related Nursing Diagnoses

ALTERATION IN NUTRITION: LESS THAN BODY REQUIREMENTS related to inability to tolerate feedings by mouth secondary to respiratory distress

INEFFECTIVE FAMILY COPING related to

a. illness of infant
b. financial difficulties of family
c. younger/older age of parents
d. single parent situation
e. location of family home (e.g., out of town)
f. lack of support system for parents/family

Medical Diagnosis	# MECONIUM ASPIRATION

Pathophysiology Meconium aspiration occurs as a consequence of fetal asphyxia. The asphyxia is thought to increase peristalsis in the intestines and relaxation of the anal sphincter, which will lead to release of meconium. The asphyxia may also cause fetal gasping, which leads to fetal aspiration of meconium. After birth, there is complete or partial airway obstruction, which decreases alveolar ventilation. The meconium lodged in the airways causes inflammation and thickening of the alveolar walls. This further impairs oxygenation, and the results are usually increased pulmonary vascular resistance and return to fetal circulation. Meconium aspiration is usually not seen in preterm infants.

Primary Nursing Diagnosis

INEFFECTIVE AIRWAY CLEARANCE

Definition Inability to clear secretions from the airways adequately

Possibly Related to Attempts by fetus to breathe in utero secondary to

- prolonged or difficult labor
- interference with the supply of oxygen via the placenta
- asphyxial episodes in utero that lead to extrauterine increase in pulmonary vascular resistance

Characteristics Tachypnea

Abnormal breath sound (i.e., crackles, rhonchi)

Cyanosis

Labored respirations (grunting and retractions)

Hypoxia

Chest x-ray revealing marked air trapping and hyperexpansion

Expected Outcomes

Infant will have an adequately clear airway as evidenced by

    a. clear and equal breath sounds bilaterally

    b. respiratory rate within the acceptable range of 30 to 60 breaths/ minute

    c. lack of cyanosis and labored respirations

    d. clear chest x-ray

Possible Nursing Interventions

- Assess and record

    —breath sounds and respiratory rate every 2 hours and PRN

    —signs/symptoms of ineffective airway clearance (such as those listed under "Characteristics") every 2 hours and PRN

    —amount and characteristics of any pulmonary secretions

- Maintain sterile technique if deep suctioning.
- Ensure that ordered oxygen is being administered in the correct amount and by the correct route. Record percentage of liter flow, route of delivery, and effectiveness of treatment.
- Ensure that chest physiotherapy is being done effectively and gently on schedule.
- Check and record results of chest x-ray when indicated.

Evaluation for Charting

- Describe breath sounds.
- State highest and lowest respiratory rates.

- Describe any signs/symptoms of ineffective airway clearance such as those listed under "Characteristics").
- Describe amount and characteristics of pulmonary secretions.
- State whether chest physiotherapy was effective in loosening secretions.
- State the results of the chest x-ray if available.

Nursing Diagnosis **IMPAIRED GAS EXCHANGE**

Definition Alteration in the exchange of oxygen and carbon dioxide in the lungs and/or at the cellular level

Possibly Related to
- Ineffective airway clearance
- Thickened alveolar walls and interstitial tissue
- Increased pulmonary vascular resistance

Characteristics Abnormal blood gas values (usually mixed respiratory and metabolic acidosis)

Hypercapnia

Hypoxemia

Cyanosis

Tachypnea

Gasping respirations

Nasal flaring

Retractions

Grunting

Expected Outcomes Infant will maintain adequate gas exchange as evidenced by

a. arterial blood gas values within acceptable range (state specific highest and lowest values for each infant)
b. respiratory rate within acceptable range of 30 to 60 breaths/minute
c. lack of

—cyanosis
—nasal flaring
—gasping respirations
—retractions
—grunting

Possible Nursing Interventions

- Assess and record every 2 hours and PRN

    —breath sounds and respiratory rate
    —signs/symptoms of impaired gas exchange (such as those listed under "Characteristics")

- Administer oxygen in correct amount and route. State effectiveness of treatment.
- If patient is intubated

    —assess patency of endotracheal tube frequently (every 30 minutes to 1 hour).
    —suction using sterile technique every 2 to 3 hours and PRN. Record amount and characteristics of secretions.
    —check ventilator settings (FiO_2, Rate, PIP or TV, PEEP/CPAP) every 15 minutes. Record every 1 to 2 hours.

Evaluation for Charting

- State highest and lowest arterial blood gas values and state the on-going physiologic process (i.e., respiratory acidosis).
- State highest and lowest respiratory rates.
- Describe any signs/symptoms of impaired gas exchange (such as those listed under "Characteristics").
- State type of endotracheal tube used and ventilator settings.

- Describe amount and characteristics of secretions.

Nursing Diagnosis **POTENTIAL FOR INFECTIONS**

Definition A condition in which the body is invaded by microorganisms

Possibly Related to
- Inflammatory response secondary to meconium
- Immature immune system

Characteristics Temperature instability
Tachypnea
Tachycardia
Lethargy
Feeding difficulties

Expected Outcomes Infant will be free of infection as evidenced by

  a. temperature between 36.5° and 37.2° C
  b. regular respiratory rate between 30 and 60 breaths/minute
  c. heart rate between 100 and 160 beats/minute
  d. lack of lethargy and feeding difficulties
  e. white blood cell count within normal limits of 9,000 to 30,000 mm³

Possible Nursing Interventions
- Assess and record every 2 hours and PRN

  —axillary temperature
  —respiratory and heart rates
  —signs/symptoms of infection (such as those listed under "Characteristics")

- Maintain neutral thermal environment.

- Ensure that antibiotics are given on schedule. Assess for any side effects such as rash or diarrhea.
- Keep accurate record of intake and output.
- Assess and record condition of IV site every hour.
- Use sterile technique when performing treatments such as suctioning and changing of IV tubing.
- Maintain good handwashing technique, especially between patients.
- Assess parents'/visitors' knowledge of handwashing technique; correct as needed.
- Check and record results of CBC.

Evaluation for Charting

- State highest and lowest body temperature and respiratory and heart rates.
- State whether a neutral thermal environment was maintained.
- Describe any signs/symptoms of infection (such as those listed under "Characteristics").
- State whether antibiotics were given on schedule. Describe any side effects.
- State intake and output.
- Describe IV site.
- State whether parents/visitors demonstrated correct handwashing technique.
- State the results of the CBC if available.

Related Nursing Diagnoses

FLUID VOLUME DEFICIT related to

a. increased insensible water loss from rapid respirations
b. lethargy

   c. fatigue

ALTERATION IN NUTRITION: LESS THAN BODY REQUIRE-MENTS related to respiratory distress

INEFFECTIVE FAMILY COPING related to serious and sudden illness of their newborn infant

Medical Diagnosis	# PERSISTENT PULMONARY HYPERTENSION OF THE NEWBORN/PERSISTENT FETAL CIRCULATION

Pathophysiology	Persistent pulmonary hypertension of the newborn (PPHN) results from pulmonary arteriolar constriction, alterations in pulmonary arterial architecture, and/or pulmonary infections. The pulmonary vasoconstriction causes high pulmonary vascular resistance and increased pulmonary artery pressure. This in turn causes the right heart pressures to become equal to or surpass systemic pressures, promoting right-to-left shunting of desaturated blood through the patent ductus arteriosus and the foramen ovale. PPHN is usually seen in term infants.

Primary Nursing Diagnosis	## IMPAIRED GAS EXCHANGE

Definition	Alteration of the exchange of oxygen and carbon dioxide in the lungs and/or at the cellular level

Possibly Related to	<ul><li>Airway obstruction secondary to aspiration of meconium</li><li>Hyperviscosity of the blood</li><li>Space-occupying lesion of the chest</li><li>Lung hypoplasia</li><li>Chronic intrauterine hypoxia</li><li>Maternal placental insufficiency</li><li>Prenatal pulmonary hypertension</li><li>Congenital heart disease</li><li>Interference with pulmonary vessel growth</li><li>Pulmonary infection</li></ul>

Characteristics   Persistent cyanosis despite attempts to
ventilate with oxygen

Tachypnea

Unequal radial and umbilical artery
blood gas values

Hypoxemia

Minimal to moderate retractions

Good air exchange on auscultation of
lungs

Normal chest x-ray

**Expected
Outcomes**   Infant will maintain adequate gas exchange as evidenced by

   a. diminished or lack of cyanosis

   b. respiratory rate within acceptable
range of 30 to 60 breaths/minute

   c. clear and equal breath sounds

   d. equal radial and umbilical artery
blood gas values

   e. arterial blood gas values within acceptable range (state specific
highest and lowest values for each
infant)

**Possible Nursing
Interventions**   • Assess and record

   —respiratory rate every 2 hours and
PRN

   —breath sounds every 2 hours and
PRN

   —signs/symptoms of impaired gas
exchange (such as those listed
under "Characteristics") every 2
hours and PRN

   —arterial blood gas values when indicated. Compare radial with umbilical values when indicated.
Notify physician if results are out
of the stated range. (Orders may
state to keep infant in respiratory

alkalosis to induce pulmonary vascular dilation).

- Ensure that oxygen is being delivered in the correct amount and by the correct route. Record percentage of liter flow and route of delivery. Assess and record effectiveness of treatment.
- Assess patency of endotracheal tube by listening to breath sounds frequently (every 30 minutes to 1 hour).
- Suction endotracheal tube using sterile technique every 2 to 3 hours and PRN. Record characteristics of secretions.
- Check ventilator settings (FiO_2, Rate, PIP or TV, PEEP/CPAP) every 15 minutes. Record every 1 to 2 hours.
- Administer vasodilators (e.g., tolazoline), smooth muscle relaxants (e.g., curare, pancuronium bromide), and volume expanders (e.g., fresh frozen plasma) on schedule if ordered. Assess and record effectiveness.
- Organize nursing care so that infant will receive minimal stimulation.

Evaluation for Charting

- State highest and lowest respiratory rates.
- Describe breath sounds and any signs/symptoms of impaired gas exchange (such as those listed under "Characteristics").
- State highest and lowest arterial blood gas values and state the on-going physiologic process (i.e., respiratory alkalosis). Note whether radial and umbilical artery blood gas values were equal.

- State amount, route, and effectiveness of oxygen therapy.
- State type of endotracheal tube and ventilator settings.
- Describe amount and characteristics of secretions.
- State whether vasodilators, smooth muscle relaxants, and/or volume expanders were administered on schedule and whether they were effective in improving gas exchange.
- State whether infant was only minimally stimulated and whether this helped improve oxygenation.

Nursing Diagnosis	**DECREASED CARDIAC OUTPUT**
Definition	A decrease in the amount of blood that leaves the left ventricle

Possibly Related to
- Hypoxemia
- Acidemia
- Systemic and pulmonary vascular pressure alterations
- Congenital heart disease

Characteristics
Systolic murmur
Poor capillary perfusion
Normal systemic blood pressure
Tachypnea
Cyanosis
Chest x-ray demonstrating mild to moderate cardiomegaly

Expected Outcomes
Infant will maintain adequate cardiac output as evidenced by

a. lack of murmur and cyanosis
b. rapid capillary refill
c. B/P within acceptable range of 64 to 96 mm Hg systolic and 30 to 62 mm Hg diastolic
d. respiratory rate within acceptable range of 30 to 60 breaths/minute

**Possible Nursing
Interventions**

e. lack of cardiomegaly on chest
x-ray

- Assess and record every 2 hours and
PRN

  —heart sounds and rate
  —B/P and respiratory rate
  —capillary refill
  —signs/symptoms of decreased cardiac output (such as those listed
  under "Characteristics")

- Check and record results of chest
x-ray if available.
- Organize nursing care so infant will
have only minimal stimulation to improve oxygenation and decrease
workload on the heart.

**Evaluation
for Charting**

- Describe heart sounds.
- State highest and lowest heart rates,
B/P, and respiratory rates.
- Describe capillary refill.
- Describe any signs/symptoms of decreased cardiac output (such as those
listed under "Characteristics").
- State results of chest x-ray if available.
- State whether infant was only minimally stimulated and whether this
helped to improve oxygenation and
cardiac output.

**Related Nursing
Diagnoses**

ALTERATION IN LEVEL OF CON-
SCIOUSNESS related to hypoxia
and acidosis
ALTERATION IN NUTRITION:
LESS THAN BODY REQUIRE-
MENTS related to decreased blood
flow to the gastrointestinal tract

FLUID VOLUME EXCESS related to hypoperfusion of the kidneys

INEFFECTIVE FAMILY COPING related to life-threatening illness of infant

Medical Diagnosis	# PNEUMONIA
Pathophysiology	Pneumonia is an infection of the lungs that can be acquired in utero (congenital pneumonia) or postnatally. The causative organism is usually bacterial in the neonate. Pneumonia is characterized by purulent exudate in the alveoli, which can lead to consolidation.
Primary Nursing Diagnosis	## INEFFECTIVE AIRWAY CLEARANCE
Definition	Inability to clear secretions from the airways adequately
Possibly Related to	An infection of the lungs caused by

- pooling of secretions secondary to prematurity
- immature immune response
- transplacental passage of microorganisms
- passage of microorganisms from infant's ascent through the birth canal
- nosocomial spread of organisms

Characteristics
Tachypnea
Abnormal breath sounds (i.e., crackles, rhonchi, wheezes)
Unequal or decreased breath sounds
Apnea
Nasal flaring
Grunting
Intercostal and subcostal retractions
Cyanosis
Tachycardia
Hypothermia or hyperthermia
Feeding difficulties
Irritability
Lethargy
Abdominal distention

Chest x-ray showing streaking infiltrates to complete consolidation

Leukocytosis or leukopenia

Expected Outcomes

Infant will have an adequately clear airway as evidenced by

    a. respiratory rate within acceptable range of 30 to 60 breaths/minute
    b. clear and equal breath sounds
    c. heart rate within acceptable range of 100 to 160 beats/minute
    d. temperature between 36.5° and 37.2° C
    e. lack of

        —nasal flaring
        —grunting
        —retractions
        —cyanosis
        —feeding difficulties
        —extreme irritability
        —extreme lethargy
        —abdominal distention

    f. clear chest x-ray
    g. white blood cell count within normal limits of 9,000 to 30,000 mm^3

Possible Nursing Interventions

• Assess and record

    —breath sounds, respiratory rate, and heart rate every 2 hours and PRN
    —signs/symptoms of ineffective airway clearance (such as those listed under "Characteristics") every 2 hours and PRN
    —amount and characteristics of any pulmonary secretions

• Maintain sterile technique when performing deep suctioning.

- Ensure that chest physiotherapy is being done effectively and gently on schedule.
- Check and record results of chest x-ray and CBC when indicated.
- Maintain good handwashing technique, especially between patients.

Evaluation for Charting

- Describe breath sounds.
- State highest and lowest respiratory and heart rates.
- Describe any signs/symptoms of ineffective airway clearance (such as those listed under "Characteristics").
- State amount, route, and effectiveness of oxygen therapy.
- Describe amount and characteristics of pulmonary secretions.
- State whether chest physiotherapy was effective in loosening secretions.
- State results of chest x-ray and CBC if available.

Nursing Diagnosis | **INEFFECTIVE THERMOREGULATION**

Definition

Instability of the infant's body temperature

Possibly Related to

Infection of the lungs (temperature is usually increased in term infants and can be decreased in premature infants)

Characteristics

Temperature instability
Increased oxygen needs
Apnea
Lethargy
Irritability

Expected Outcomes

Infant will maintain effective thermoregulation as evidenced by

a. temperature within acceptable range of 36.5° to 37.2° C
b. stable oxygen needs

c. lack of

—apnea
—extreme lethargy
—extreme irritability

Possible Nursing Interventions

- Assess and record every 2 hours and PRN

  —infant's axillary temperature
  —signs/symptoms of temperature instability (such as those listed under "Characteristics")

- Ensure that a neutral thermal environment is maintained. Note changes in ambient temperature, skin temperature, and heater output as related to axillary temperature.
- Always use alarms and skin probes when using infant warmers and isolettes.
- Place plastic sheet or bubble bag over infants in open warmers when indicated.
- Keep infant away from air drafts.
- Prewarm any surface on which infant is placed, such as an x-ray plate.
- Keep infant dry. Change as soon as possible after elimination.

Evaluation for Charting

- State highest and lowest axillary temperature.
- Describe any signs/symptoms of ineffective thermoregulation (such as those listed under "Characteristics").
- Describe any successful methods used to help prevent ineffective thermoregulation.
- State whether a neutral thermal environment was maintained.
- State whether oxygen needs were stable.

Related Nursing Diagnoses

ALTERATION IN COMFORT related to chest pain

FLUID VOLUME DEFICIT related to increased insensible water loss from rapid respirations

ALTERATION IN NUTRITION: LESS THAN BODY REQUIREMENTS related to

a. feeding difficulties
b. abdominal distention
c. lethargy

INEFFECTIVE FAMILY COPING related to increased length of hospital stay for infant

| Medical Diagnosis | **PNEUMOTHORAX** |

Pathophysiology

A pneumothorax is an accumulation of air (or blood) in the pleural space that destroys the negative pressure and causes the lung to collapse. It can be spontaneous or occur as a complication of assisted ventilation, pulmonary disease, or certain procedures. Diagnosis can be made by transillumination of the chest and confirmed by chest x-ray. Treatment can include the administration of 100% oxygen ("nitrogen washout technique," which could be used with a term infant in mild respiratory distress), needle aspiration of the chest, or the insertion of a chest tube.

Primary Nursing Diagnosis

IMPAIRED GAS EXCHANGE

Definition

Alteration in the exchange of oxygen and carbon dioxide in the lungs and/or at the cellular level

Possibly Related to

Collapsed lung (or collapsed portion of a lung) secondary to

- fetal distress
- difficult delivery
- aspiration of meconium
- lung infection
- high ventilator pressure
- zealous bag ventilation

Characteristics

Tachypnea
Grunting
Nasal flaring
Retractions
Cyanosis
Diminished breath sounds on the affected side
Agitation irritability

Increasing oxygen or ventilator needs

Transillumination of the chest revealing air pockets

Chest x-ray revealing air pockets (dark area along the edge of the affected lung)

ADVANCED STAGES

Apnea

Bradycardia (initially heart rate is increased)

Drop in blood pressure (initially blood pressure is increased)

Mediastinal shift

Decreased pulse pressure

Expected Outcomes

Infant will maintain adequate gas exchange as evidenced by

a. respiratory rate within acceptable range of 30 to 60 breaths/minute
b. lack of

—grunting
—nasal flaring
—retractions
—cyanosis
—extreme agitation/irritability
—apnea

c. clear and equal breath sounds
d. arterial blood gas values within acceptable range (state specific highest and lowest values for each infant)
e. no visible air pocket on transillumination
f. clear chest x-ray
g. heart rate within acceptable range of 100 to 160 beats/minute
h. blood pressure within acceptable range of 64/30 to 96/62 mm Hg
i. midline mediastinum

j. pulse pressure within acceptable limits of 20 to 50 mm Hg

Possible Nursing Interventions

- Assess and record

    —respiratory rate, heart rate, blood pressure, and breath sounds every 2 hours and PRN
    —position of mediastinum every 2 hours and PRN
    —arterial blood gas values when indicated. Notify physician if results are out of the stated range.
    —any signs/symptoms of impaired gas exchange (such as those listed under "Characteristics") every 2 hours and PRN

- Ensure that oxygen is being delivered in the correct amount and by the correct route. Record percentage of liter flow and route of delivery. Assess and record effectiveness of treatment.
- Assess patency of endotracheal tube by listening to breath sounds frequently (every 30 minutes to 1 hour).
- Suction endotracheal tube using sterile technique every 2 to 3 hours and PRN. Record amount and characteristics of secretions.
- Check ventilator settings (FiO2, Rate, PIP or TV, PEEP/CPAP) every 15 minutes. Record every 1 to 2 hours.
- Prepare infant for any medical treatment such as needle aspiration or the insertion of chest tubes. Record infant's tolerance and the effectiveness of any indicated procedures.

- Explain any procedure and the rationale for doing the procedure to the infant's family.
- Check and record results of chest x-ray and transillumination of the chest when indicated.
- Ensure that chest physiotherapy is being done gently and effectively on schedule. Record infant's response and effectiveness of treatment.
- Reposition infant every 2 hours.
- If a chest tube is inserted

  —assess and record amount and characteristics of drainage every shift and PRN (usually a total of 3 to 5 ml/shift)
  —assess amount of bubbling hourly. Count and record the number of bubbles for 1 minute every shift.
  —keep a hemostat or clamp at the bedside to clamp the tube if the system becomes disconnected
  —gently milk chest tubes (if ordered) every 4 hours
  —keep petrolatum gauze at the bedside to apply to the wound site in case the chest tube becomes dislodged

Evaluation for Charting

- State highest and lowest respiratory rate, heart rate, and blood pressure.
- Describe breath sounds and position of mediastinum.
- Describe any signs/symptoms of impaired gas exchange (such as those listed under "Characteristics").
- State highest and lowest arterial blood gas values and state the on-going physiologic process (i.e., respiratory acidosis).

- State type of endotracheal tube in place and ventilator settings.
- Describe amount and characteristics of secretions.
- Describe the effectiveness of and infant's tolerance to any therapeutic measures used to improve gas exchange.
- Describe the results of transillumination and/or chest x-ray if indicated.
- State whether the chest physiotherapy treatments were effective in improving gas exchange.
- State whether the infant was repositioned every 2 hours.
- Describe the amount and characteristics of chest drainage.
- State the number of bubbles present per minute in the water seal chamber.

Nursing Diagnosis **DECREASED CARDIAC OUTPUT**

Definition A decrease in the amount of blood that leaves the left ventricle

Possibly Related to Characteristics

Impaired venous return to the heart
Bradycardia
Decreased blood pressure
Mediastinal shift
Shift in the point of maximal impulse of the heart
Decreased pulse pressure
Cyanosis

Expected Outcomes

Infant will maintain adequate cardiac output as evidenced by

a. heart rate within acceptable range of 100 to 160 beats/minute
b. blood pressure within acceptable range of 64/30 to 96/62 mm Hg

c. midline mediastinum and appropriate location for the point of maximal impulse of the heart

d. pulse pressure within acceptable limits of 20 to 50 mm Hg

e. lack of cyanosis

Possible Nursing Interventions

- Assess and record every 2 hours and PRN

  —heart rate and blood pressure

  —position of mediastinum and point of maximal impulse

  —signs/symptoms of decreased cardiac output (such as those listed under "Characteristics")

- Organize nursing care to allow rest periods to decrease workload on the heart.

- Elevate head of bed at a 30° angle.

Evaluation for Charting

- State highest and lowest heart rate and blood pressure.

- Describe position of mediastinum and point of maximal impulse.

- Describe any signs/symptoms of decreased cardiac output (such as those listed under "Characteristics").

- State whether head of bed was elevated.

Related Nursing Diagnoses

ALTERATION IN COMFORT related to pain on affected side

POTENTIAL FOR INFECTION related to invasive procedures

FLUID VOLUME DEFICIT related to inability to tolerate fluids by mouth secondary to respiratory distress

INEFFECTIVE FAMILY COPING related to

a. illness of infant
b. need for additional invasive procedures

Medical Diagnosis	# PULMONARY INTERSTITIAL EMPHYSEMA
Pathophysiology	Pulmonary interstitial emphysema (PIE) occurs when air is interposed between the alveoli and the capillaries that surround them. It can occur after barotrauma secondary to ventilatory management. Impairment of gas exchange and circulation results. Management usually includes increased mechanical ventilator and oxygen settings. Diagnosis can be made by x-ray examination. If PIE is present, the x-ray will reveal small, dark, air-filled pockets within the lung tissue. Progression to pneumothorax occurs frequently.
Primary Nursing Diagnosis	## IMPAIRED GAS EXCHANGE
Definition	Alteration in the exchange of oxygen and carbon dioxide in the lungs and/or at the cellular level
Possibly Related to	• Air leaks from the base of the alveoli into the interstitial perivascular space • Positive airway pressure supplied by a ventilator and/or CPAP • Barotrauma secondary to ventilatory management
Characteristics	Tachypnea Retractions Increasing oxygen needs Need to increase pressure and rate settings on mechanical ventilator Deterioration of arterial blood gas values Color changes such as cyanosis or mottling Irritability

Restlessness

Chest x-ray revealing small, dark, air-filled pockets within the lung tissue

Expected Outcomes

Infant will maintain adequate gas exchange as evidenced by

a. respiratory rate within acceptable range of 30 to 60 breaths/minute
b. stable oxygen needs
c. stable ventilatory settings
d. arterial blood gas values within acceptable range (state specific highest and lowest values for each infant)
e. lack of

—cyanosis or mottling
—retractions
—extreme irritability
—extreme restlessness

f. clear chest x-ray

Possible Nursing Interventions

• Assess and record

—respiratory rate and breath sounds every 2 hours and PRN
—signs/symptoms of impaired gas exchange (such as those listed under "Characteristics") every 2 hours and PRN
—arterial blood gas values when indicated. Notify physician if results are out of the stated range.

• Ensure that oxygen is being delivered in the correct amount and by the correct route. Record percentage of liter flow and route of delivery. Assess and record effectiveness of treatment.

- Assess patency of endotracheal tube by listening to breath sounds frequently (every 30 minutes to 1 hour).
- Suction endotracheal tube using sterile technique every 2 to 3 hours and PRN. Record amount and characteristics of secretions.
- Check ventilator settings (FiO_2, Rate, PIP or TV, PEEP/CPAP) every 15 minutes. Record every 1 to 2 hours.
- Transilluminate infant's chest every 2 to 4 hours while on ventilator if indicated. Record results.
- Prepare infant for any medical treatment such as needle aspiration or insertion of chest tubes.
- Explain any procedure and the rationale for doing the procedure to the infant's family.
- Check and record results of chest x-ray when indicated.

Evaluation for Charting

- Describe breath sounds.
- State highest and lowest respiratory rates.
- Describe any signs/symptoms of impaired gas exchange (such as those listed under "Characteristics").
- State highest and lowest arterial blood gas values and state the on-going physiologic process (i.e., respiratory acidosis).
- State type of endotracheal tube in place and ventilator settings.
- Describe amount and characteristics of secretions.
- Describe the effectiveness of and infant's tolerance to any therapeutic measures used to improve gas exchange.

- Describe results of transillumination.
- Describe results of chest x-ray if available.

Nursing Diagnosis **DECREASED CARDIAC OUTPUT**

Definition A decrease in the amount of blood that leaves the left ventricle

Possibly Related to Circulatory impairment secondary to vessel compression

Characteristics Tachycardia
Tachypnea
Hypotension
Cyanosis
Feeding difficulties
Fatigue

Expected Outcomes Infant will maintain adequate cardiac output as evidenced by

 a. heart rate within acceptable range of 100 to 160 beats/minute
 b. respiratory rate within acceptable range of 30 to 60 breaths/minute
 c. blood pressure within acceptable range of 64/30 to 96/62 mm Hg
 d. lack of

  —cyanosis
  —fatigue
  —feeding difficulties

Possible Nursing Interventions

- Assess and record every 2 hours and PRN

 —heart and respiratory rates
 —blood pressure
 —signs/symptoms of decreased cardiac output (such as those listed under "Characteristics")

- Organize nursing care to allow rest periods to decrease workload on the heart.

Evaluation for Charting

- Elevate head of bed at a 30° angle.

- State highest and lowest heart and respiratory rates.
- State highest and lowest B/P.
- Describe any signs/symptoms of decreased cardiac output (such as those listed under "Characteristics").
- State whether head of bed was elevated.

Related Nursing Diagnoses

POTENTIAL FOR INFECTION related to

a. surgical puncture wound
b. insertion of chest tube
c. immature immune system

ALTERATION IN NUTRITION: LESS THAN BODY REQUIREMENTS related to inability to tolerate feedings by mouth secondary to respiratory distress

INEFFECTIVE FAMILY COPING related to

a. illness of infant
b. need for additional invasive procedures

PARENTAL KNOWLEDGE DEFICIT related to new complication of disease process

Medical Diagnosis	# TRANSIENT TACHYPNEA OF THE NEWBORN
Pathophysiology	Transient tachypnea of the newborn (TTN) is a persistently high respiratory rate, usually transient, that occurs in term or near-term infants. It is generally self-limiting (resolving in a few days) and thought to be secondary to slow absorption of normal lung fluid. The result is diffuse emphysema and air trapping with mild hypoxemia and acidemia. TTN may also be referred to as respiratory distress syndrome II (RDS II).
Primary Nursing Diagnosis	## INEFFECTIVE BREATHING PATTERN
Definition	A breathing pattern that results in oxygen insufficient to meet the cellular requirements of the body
Possibly Related to Characteristics	Delay in absorption of fetal lung fluid Tachypnea (usually in excess of 80 breaths/minute) Minimal retractions Flaring of the nostrils Expiratory grunt Minimal or no cyanosis Mild hypoxemia Mild acidemia Good air exchange X-ray characterized by generalized overexpansion, central peripheral streaking, flattened diaphragm, and increased AP diameter
Expected Outcomes	Infant will maintain an effective breathing pattern as evidenced by

   a. respiratory rate within acceptable range of 30 to 60 breaths/minute

b. clear and equal breath sounds
c. lack of

  —retractions
  —nasal flaring
  —expiratory grunt
  —cyanosis

d. arterial blood gas values within acceptable range (state specific highest and lowest values for each infant)
e. normal chest x-ray

Possible Nursing Interventions

- Assess and record

  —respiratory rate every 2 hours and PRN
  —breath sounds every 2 hours and PRN
  —signs/symptoms of ineffective breathing pattern (such as those listed under "Characteristics") every 2 hours and PRN
  —arterial blood gas values when indicated

- Ensure that oxygen (usually less than 40%) is being delivered in the correct amount and route. Record percentage of liter flow and route of delivery every 2 hours. State effectiveness of treatment.

Evaluation for Charting

- State highest and lowest respiratory rates.
- Describe breath sounds and any signs/symptoms of ineffective breathing pattern (such as those listed under "Characteristics").
- State highest and lowest arterial blood gas values and state the on-going physiologic process (i.e., respiratory acidosis).

- State amount, route, and effectiveness of oxygen therapy.

Nursing Diagnosis

FLUID VOLUME DEFICIT

Definition

A decrease in the amount of circulating fluid volume

Possibly Related to

- Insensible water loss from rapid respirations
- Inability to tolerate fluids by mouth

Characteristics

Tachypnea
Sunken fontanel
Sunken eyes
Poor skin turgor
Dry mucous membranes
Decreased urinary output

Expected Outcomes

Child will maintain adequate fluid volume as evidenced by

a. adequate amount of IV fluids (state specific amount of intake needed for each infant)
b. flat fontanel
c. normal orbital contour
d. rapid skin recoil
e. moist mucous membrances
f. adequate urinary output (state acceptable minimal urinary output—0.5 to 1 ml/kg/hour)
g. urine specific gravity of 1.008 to 1.020

Possible Nursing Interventions

- Keep accurate record of intake and output.
- Weigh diapers for urine output.
- Assess and record

—IV fluids and condition of IV site every hour
—signs/symptoms of fluid volume deficit (such as those listed under

"Characteristics") every 2 to 4
hours and PRN.

- Check and record urine specific gravity every void or as directed.

**Evaluation
for Charting**

- State intake and output.
- Describe condition of IV site.
- Describe any signs/symptoms of fluid volume deficit (such as those listed under "Characteristics").
- State highest and lowest urine specific gravity.

**Related Nursing
Diagnoses**

ALTERATION IN NUTRITION: LESS THAN BODY REQUIREMENTS related to

a. inability to tolerate feedings by mouth secondary to rapid respirations

b. increased utilization of glucose during stress

INEFFECTIVE FAMILY COPING, related to unexpected illness of newborn (usually term infant)

PARENTAL KNOWLEDGE DEFICIT related to unexpected illness of term newborn

INEFFECTIVE THERMOREGULATION related to increased metabolic rate

PATENT DUCTUS ARTERIOSUS

Pathophysiology

The ductus arteriosus is a connection between the pulmonary artery and the aorta. In utero, the ductus arteriosus provides a means of shunting blood away from the pulmonary circuit into the systemic circulation via the descending aorta. The ductus is composed of smooth muscle and elastic tissue. When oxygen is present in sufficient amounts, it acts directly on the smooth muscle cells of the ductus and causes it to constrict. Insufficient oxygenation results in continued patency of the ductus arteriosus. Patency of the ductus arteriosus leads to a left-top-right cardiac shunt resulting in decreased oxygenated blood flow to the systemic circulation and increased blood flow under increased pressure to the lungs. This hyperperfusion of the lungs along with greater capillary permeability causes pulmonary edema and can lead to congestive heart failure.

Primary Nursing Diagnosis

IMPAIRED GAS EXCHANGE

Definition

Alteration in the exchange of oxygen and carbon dioxide in the lungs and/or at the cellular level

Possibly Related to

Patent fetal circulatory opening between the pulmonary artery and the aorta secondary to hypoxemia and poorly developed ductal muscle wall

Characteristics

Tachypnea
Expiratory grunt
Intercostal retractions
Crackles
Hypercarbia

Hypoxemia

Difference between gases in radial artery and umbilical artery

Expected Outcomes

Infant will maintain adequate gas exchange as evidenced by

   a. respiratory rate within acceptable range of 30 to 60 breaths/minute

   b. lack of

      —expiratory grunt
      —retractions

   c. clear and equal breath sounds

   d. arterial blood gas values within acceptable range (state specific highest and lowest values for each infant)

   e. relatively equal (within 10 mm Hg) gases in radial artery and umbilical artery

Possible Nursing Interventions

• Assess and record

   —respiratory rate and breath sounds every 2 hours and PRN

   —signs/symptoms of impaired gas exchange (such as those listed under "Characteristics") every 2 hours and PRN

   —arterial blood gas values when indicated. Notify physician if results are out of the stated range.

• Ensure that oxygen is being delivered in the correct amount and by the correct route. Record percentage of liter flow and route of delivery. Assess and record effectiveness of treatment.

• If infant is intubated, check ventilator settings (FiO2, Rate, PIP or TV, PEEP/CPAP) every 15 minutes. Record every 1 to 2 hours. Suction using sterile technique every 2 hours and PRN. Record amount and characteristics of secretions.

Evaluation for Charting
- State highest and lowest respiratory rates.
- Describe breath sounds.
- Describe any signs/symptoms of impaired gas exchange (such as those listed under "Characteristics").
- State highest and lowest arterial blood gas values and state the no-going physiologic process (i.e., respiratory acidosis). Compare radial and umbilical artery values.
- State amount and route of oxygen delivery. Describe effectiveness.
- State type of endotracheal tube used and ventilator settings.
- State frequency of suctioning and describe amount and characteristics of secretions.

Nursing Diagnosis

DECREASED CARDIAC OUTPUT

Definition
A decrease in the amount of blood that leaves the left ventricle

Possibly Related to
- Cardiac defect
- Increased blood flow under increased pressure to the lungs
- Increased workload on the right side of the heart

Characteristics
Tachycardia
Machinery-like systolic murmur
Wide pulse pressure
Bounding peripheral pulses
Heavy percordial impulse (hyperactive precordium)
Hepatomegaly
Edema

Expected Outcomes   Infant will maintain adequate cardiac output as evidenced by

    a. heart rate within acceptable range of 100 to 160 beats/minute

    b. pulse pressure within acceptable limits of 20 to 50 mm Hg

    c. strong (nonbounding) peripheral pulses

    d. lack of

      —murmur
      —hyperactive precordium
      —hepatomegaly
      —edema

    e. adequate urinary output (state acceptable minimal urinary output, 0.5 to 1 ml/kg/hour)

Possible Nursing Interventions

- Assess and record

    —heart rate and blood pressure every 2 hours and PRN

    —position of liver every 8 hours and PRN

    —signs/symptoms of decreased cardiac output (such as those listed under "Characteristics") every 2 hours and PRN

- Organize nursing care to allow rest periods to decrease workload on the heart.
- Administer indomethacin if ordered. Assess and record effectiveness and any side effects (such as edema, impaired renal and hepatic function).
- Keep accurate record of intake and output.
- If indicated, prepare infant and family for surgery (ligation of patent ductus arteriosus).

Evaluation for Charting

- State highest and lowest heart rates and blood pressure.
- Describe position of liver.
- Describe any signs/symptoms of decreased cardiac output (such as those listed under "Characteristics").
- State whether indomethacin was administered on schedule. Describe effectiveness (if possible) and any side effects.
- State intake and output.

Related Nursing Diagnoses

FLUID VOLUME EXCESS related to

a. cardiac defect
b. increased flow under increased pressure to the lungs
c. increased workload on the right side of the heart
d. decreased blood flow to the kidneys
e. side effect of medication (indomethacin)

ALTERATION IN NUTRITION: LESS THAN BODY REQUIREMENTS related to hypoxemia and decreased blood flow to the gastointestinal tract

INEFFECTIVE THERMOREGULATION related to hypoxemia and acidosis

INEFFECTIVE FAMILY COPING related to

a. defect of a major organ
b. increased time of hospital stay for infant
c. possible need for surgery

Medical Diagnosis

NECROTIZING ENTEROCOLITIS

Pathophysiology

Necrotizing enterocolitis (NEC) is a septic necrosis of the mucosa or submucosa of the small and/or large bowel. It can be diffuse or patchy. Initially the necrosis may be localized, but it can spread, leading to bowel perforation or infarction. The cause of NEC is uncertain. Current theory suggests that the immature infant responds to perinatal stress and hypoxia by shunting too much blood to the vital organs, thus reducing mesenteric circulation.

There are many predisposing risk factors for NEC. Prematurity is the greatest risk factor, with 80 to 90% of cases diagnosed in infants weighing less than 2500 grams. Other risk factors include perinatal asphyxia, respiratory distress syndrome, umbilical catheterization, hypothermia, hypotension, hypoxia, patent ductus arteriosus, cyanotic heart disease, polycythemia, thrombocytosis, anemia, exchange transfusions, thrombosis, emboli, vasospasm, diet of non-breast milk formula, ingestion of too much formula too fast, hospitalization during epidemic, direct bacterial invasion, and bacterial overgrowth.

The onset of NEC may be sudden and rapid or slow with variable intensity. Treatment is aimed at resting the bowel and managing complications. Surgery is necessary if deterioration continues 72 hours after treatment has been initiated or if the bowel is perforated.

Primary Nursing Diagnosis	**ALTERATION IN NUTRITION: LESS THAN BODY REQUIREMENTS**
Definition	Insufficient nutrients to meet body needs
Possibly Related to	• Decreased perfusion to the gastrointestinal tract • Hypoxia • Non-breast milk formula feedings • Hypertonic feedings • Polycythemia • Vasospasm • Complication of umbilical catheterization • Direct bacterial invasion
Characteristics	*Systemic* Temperature instability Lethargy Apnea Bradycardia Failure to gain weight Decreased blood platelets *Abdominal* Abdominal distention Inability to tolerate feedings Faint or absent bowel sounds Erythema at umbilicus Bile-stained, coffee-ground, or bloody vomitus Positive stool tests for blood and reducing sugars Abdominal x-ray revealing dilated loops of intestine and gas bubbles in the wall of the intestine
Expected Outcomes	Infant will be free of signs/symptoms of nutritional deficit as evidenced by a. temperature between 36.5° and 37.2° C

b. heart rate within acceptable range of 100 to 160 beats/minute
c. weight gain of 10 to 20 grams/day
d. platelet count between 100,000 and 400,000 cells/mm^3
e. absence of abdominal distention: stable abdominal girth
f. ability to tolerate feedings
g. minimal (2 to 3 ml) to no residual gastric contents before tube feeding
h. active bowel sounds
i. lack of

   —apnea
   —extreme lethargy
   —erythema around umbilicus
   —blood or reducing sugars in stool

j. abdominal x-ray negative for distended loops of intestine and visible gas bubbles in the wall of the intestines
k. weight gain of 10 to 20 grams/day

Possible Nursing Interventions
- Assess and record

  —temperature and heart rate every 2 hours and PRN
  —abdominal distention every shift; measure and record abdominal girth every shift and PRN
  —bowel sounds every shift
  —signs/symptoms of nutritional deficit/necrotizing enterocolitis (such as those listed under "Characteristics") every 2 hours and PRN

- Weigh daily on same scale at same time of day without clothes.
- Keep accurate record of intake and output including gastric residual contents before tube feeding.

- Test stools for blood and reducing sugars when indicated. Record results.
- Provide oral care every shift if infant is NPO.
- Assess nasogastric tube for position and patency every 2 hours. Connect it to low intermittent suction or gravity drainage as ordered. Record characteristics of any drainage.
- Assess area around umbilicus every 4 hours. Record results and notify physician of any abnormalities.

Evaluation for Charting

- State highest and lowest temperature and heart rate.
- Describe abdominal assessment.
- State abdominal girth and indicate whether it has increased, decreased, or remained the same as the previous measurement.
- Describe any signs/symptoms of nutritional deficit/necrotizing enterocolitis (such as those listed under "Characteristics").
- State intake and output including gastric residual contents.
- State current weight and determine whether it has increased or decreased since last weighing.
- State results of tests for blood or reducing sugars in stools when indicated.
- State whether nasogastric tube was patent and in place. Describe characteristics of any drainage.
- Describe area around umbilicus.

Nursing Diagnosis **INEFFECTIVE BREATHING PATTERN**

Definition A breathing pattern that results in oxygen insufficient to meet the cellular requirements of the body

Possibly Related to
- Abdominal distention
- Hypoxia

Characteristics
Tachypnea
Apnea
Retractions
Nasal flaring

Expected Outcomes

Infant will maintain an effective breathing pattern as evidenced by

a. respiratory rate within acceptable range of 30 to 60 breaths/minute
b. clear and equal breath sounds
c. lack of

—apnea
—retractions
—nasal flaring

Possible Nursing Interventions
- Assess and record every 2 hours and PRN

—respiratory rate and breath sounds
—signs/symptoms of ineffective breathing pattern (such as those listed under "Characteristics")

- Ensure that oxygen is being delivered in the correct amount and by the correct route. Record percentage of liter flow and route of delivery every 2 hours. State effectiveness of treatment.

Evaluation for Charting
- State highest and lowest respiratory rates.
- Describe breath sounds.
- Describe any signs/symptoms of ineffective breathing pattern (such as those listed under "Characteristics").
- State amount, route, and effectiveness of oxygen therapy.

DECREASED CARDIAC OUTPUT related to

    a. hypoxia

    b. polycythemia

    c. bleeding from the gastrointestinal tract

    d. decreased platelets

FLUID VOLUME DEFICIT related to

    a. vomiting

    b. bleeding from the gastrointestinal tract

INFECTION related to

    a. bacterial invasion of the gastrointestinal tract

    b. additional invasive procedures

    c. possibility of surgery for bowel resection

| Medical Diagnosis | # OMPHALOCELE/ GASTROSCHISIS |

Pathophysiology

An omphalocele is a congenital malformation in which there is protrusion of abdominal contents into the base of the umbilical cord. This is normally where the viscera is located in early embryonic life (the sixth to the tenth week). After the tenth week of fetal life, the abdominal cavity should be large enough to accommodate the abdominal contents. When an omphalocele occurs, the abdominal cavity is generaly underdeveloped and the intestines and liver fail to return to the abdominal cavity. The defect can be large or small and is commonly associated with cardiovascular, genitourinary, or other gastrointestinal problems. The defect is surgically repaired (closed). If it is not possible to do a primary repair, the defect is covered (with silicone-coated mesh) and reduced gradually over 7 to 10 days.

Gastroschisis is a defect in the abdominal wall that allows abdominal contents to protrude outside the body. This defect is located to the right of the umbilicus. The exposed contents can range from the stomach to the rectum. Unlike an omphalocele, a gastroschisis has no sac covering the exposed contents. Some refer to gastroschisis as a "ruptured omphalocele." Surgical correction of the defect should be done as soon as the infant's condition is stabilized. This surgery can be done in a one-stage operation (80%) or may need to be a multistage reduction repair (10%).

Preoperative

Primary Nursing Diagnosis **POTENTIAL FOR INFECTION**

Definition Invasion of the body by pathogenic organisms

Possibly Related to Protrusion of unprotected abdominal contents

Characteristics Temperature instability
Tachypnea
Lethargy
Hypotonia

Expected Outcomes Infant will be free of infection as evidenced by

a. temperature between 36.5° and 37.2° C
b. respiratory rate within acceptable range of 30 to 60 breaths/minute
c. lack of
—lethargy
—hypotonia
d. white blood cell count within normal limits of 9,000 to 30,000 mm^3

Possible Nursing Interventions

- Assess and record
  —axillary temperature and respiratory rate every 2 hours and PRN
  —signs/symptoms of infection (such as those listed under "Characteristics") every 4 hours and PRN
- Maintain a neutral thermal environment.
- Ensure that a sterile moist dressing is maintained on sac or exposed viscera.
- Keep accurate record of intake and output.
- Ensure that antibiotics are given on schedule. Assess and record effec-

tiveness and any side effects (such as diarrhea or rash).
- Maintain good handwashing technique.
- Check and record results of CBC. Notify physician if CBC results are out of the acceptable range.

Evalutation for Charting
- State highest and lowest axillary temperature and respiratory rate.
- Describe any signs/symptoms of infection (such as those listed under "Characteristics").
- State whether a neutral thermal environment was maintained.
- State whether a sterile moist dressing was maintained on the sac or exposed viscera?
- State intake and output.
- State whether antibiotics were administered on schedule. Describe effectiveness and any side effects.
- State whether good handwashing technique was maintained.
- State results of CBC, if available.

Nursing Diagnosis
INEFFECTIVE THERMOREGULATION

Definition
Instability of the infant's body temperature

Possibly Related to Characteristics
Added exposed surface area
Temperature instability
Increased oxygen needs
Lethargy
Apnea
Bradycardia

Expected Outcomes
Infant will maintain effective thermoregulation as evidenced by

a. temperature within acceptable range of 36.5° to 37.2° C

b. stable oxygen needs
c. lack of lethargy
d. lack of apnea
e. heart rate within acceptable range of 100 to 160 beats/minute

Possible Nursing Interventions

• Assess and record

—infant's axillary temperature and heart rate every 2 hours and PRN
—signs/symptoms of temperature instability (such as those listed under "Characteristics") every 4 hours and PRN

• Ensure that a neutral thermal environment is maintained. Note changes in ambient temperature, skin temperature, and heater output as related to axillary temperature.
• Always use alarms and skin probes when using infant warmers and isolettes.
• Place plastic sheet or bubble bag over infants in open warmers when indicated.
• Keep infant away from air drafts.
• Prewarm any surface on which infant is to be placed, such as an x-ray plate.
• Keep infant dry. Change as soon as possible after elimination.

Evaluation for Charting

• State highest and lowest axillary temperature and heart rate.
• Describe any signs/symptoms of ineffective thermoregulation (such as those listed under "Characteristics").
• Describe any successful methods used to help prevent ineffective thermoregulation.
• State whether a neutral thermal environment was maintained.

- State whether oxygen needs were stable.

Related Nursing Diagnoses

FLUID DEFICIT AND ELECTRO-LYTE IMBALANCE related to

a. exposed viscera before surgical repair
b. excessive heat loss
c. third spacing of fluid
d. nasogastric suctioning

ALTERATION IN NUTRITION: LESS THAN BODY REQUIRE-MENTS related to

a. inability of infant to tolerate feedings by mouth
b. delayed intestinal motility secondary to prolonged exposure of the intestines to amniotic fluid

INEFFECTIVE FAMILY COPING related to obvious physical anomaly and severity of illness (40% mortality rate with gastroschisis)

PARENTAL KNOWLEDGE DEFI-CIT related to uncommonness of defect (1 in 3000 to 5000 for omphalocele and 1 in 50,000 for gastroschisis)

Postoperative

Primary Nursing Diagnosis

INEFFECTIVE BREATHING PATTERN

Definition

A breathing pattern that results in oxgen insufficient to meet the cellular requirements of the body

Possibly Related to

Increased pressure on the diaphragm secondary to placement of abdominal contents into the abdominal cavity

Characteristics

Tachypnea
Retractions

Nasal flaring
Atelectasis

Expected Outcomes

Infant will maintain an effective breathing pattern as evidenced by

    a. respiratory rate within acceptable range of 30 to 60 breaths/minute
    b. lack of

      —retractions
      —nasal flaring

    c. clear chest x-ray
    d. clear and equal breath sounds bilaterally

Possible Nursing Interventions

- Assess and record

    —respiratory rate every 2 hours and PRN
    —breath sounds
    —signs/symptoms of ineffective breathing pattern (such as those listed under "Characteristics") every 2 hours and PRN

- Ensure that nasogastric tube is in place (to decompress the stomach and prevent aspiration).
- Elevate head of bed at a 30° angle.
- Reposition infant every 2 hours unless contraindicated.
- Ensure that chest physiotherapy is being done gently and effectively on schedule. Record effectiveness of treatment.

Evaluation for Charting

- State highest and lowest respiratory rate.
- Describe breath sounds.
- Describe any signs/symptoms of ineffective breathing pattern (such as those listed under "Characteristics").

- State whether the nasogastric tube was positioned correctly and whether it was effective in decompressing the stomach.
- State whether the head of the bed was elevated at a 30° angle.
- State whether the infant was repositioned every 2 hours.
- Describe the effectiveness of chest physiotherapy.

Nursing Diagnosis	**DECREASED CARDIAC OUTPUT**
Definition	A decrease in the amount of blood that leaves the left ventricle
Possibly Related to	Pressure of the vena cava secondary to placement of abdominal contents into the abdominal cavity
Characteristics	Peripheral edema
	Prolonged capillary refill, longer than 2 to 3 seconds
	Decreased or unequal peripheral pulses
	Tachycardia
	Tachypnea
Expected Outcomes	Infant will maintain adequate cardiac output as evidenced by

a. lack of edema
b. brisk capillary refill, within 2 to 3 seconds
c. strong and equal peripheral pulses
d. heart rate within acceptable range of 100 to 160 beats/minute
e. respiratory rate within acceptable range of 30 to 60 breaths/minute

Possible Nursing Interventions

- Assess and record every 2 hours and PRN

—evidence of edema (amount and location)
—capillary refill
—peripheral pulses
—heart rate and respiratory rate
- Keep accurate record of intake and output.
- Elevate head of bed at a 30° angle.

Evaluation for Charting

- Describe amount and location of edema.
- Describe capillary refill.
- Describe quality of peripheral pulses.
- State highest and lowest heart rate and respiratory rate.
- State intake and output.
- State whether head of bed was maintained at a 30° angle?

Related Nursing Diagnoses

POTENTIAL FOR INFECTION related to invasive procedures

ALTERATION IN COMFORT related to

a. surgical intervention
b. hunger pangs (maintained on IV therapy)
c. gas accumulation before return of peristalsis

ALTERATION IN NUTRITION: LESS THAN BODY REQUIREMENTS related to possible bowel necrosis from excessive organ crowding

INEFFECTIVE FAMILY COPING related to

a. separation from newborn
b. needed surgical intervention
c. possibility of long-term treatment and rehabilitation

HYPERBILIRUBINEMIA

Pathophysiology

Hyperbilirubinemia or jaundice is common in infants, occurring in 50% of term infants and 80% of premature infants. If adult standards were used, all neonates would be considered to have hyperbilirubinemia (bilirubin exceeding 1 mg/100ml). Bilirubin results from the breakdown of red blood cells. Jaundice is an increase of the bilirubin due to overproduction of bilirubin or deficient conjugation of bilirubin.

Physiologic jaundice, which is temporary and normal, can occur in term infants around the third day of life with indirect (unconjugated) bilirubin levels of up to 12 mg/100 ml. The level decreases gradually to normal by 10 days of age. Premature infants who have physiologic jaundice can have direct bilirubin levels of 12 mg/100 ml by the fifth day of life. The causes of physiologic jaundice are controversial. Factors contributing to neonatal jaundice are that the newborn has more red blood cells than an adult and that the life span of an infant's red blood cells is shorter. Pathologic jaundice occurs within the first 36 hours of life and is usually the result of overproduction of bilirubin.

Increased levels of indirect bilirubin can be caused by isoimmunization from blood type or Rh incompatibility between mother and baby, hereditary spherocytosis, birth trauma causing hemorrhage or bleeding, polycythemia, or hypothyroidism. Elevation of direct or conjugated bilirubin can result from sepsis, biliary atresia, neonatal hepatitis, and prolonged hyperalimentation. Kernicterus, a complication of hyperbilirubinemia, occurs when there are toxic levels of bilirubin in the brain tissue.

Primary Nursing Diagnosis

ALTERATION IN METABOLIC FUNCTION

Definition Imbalance in the body's utilization of specific biochemicals

Possibly Related to

- Overproduction of bilirubin
- Impaired excretion of bilirubin
- Deficient conjugation of bilirubin

Characteristics Jaundice
Lethargy
Feeding difficulties
Edema
Ascites
Dark urine
Clay-colored stools
Pruritus
Seizures
High-pitched cry

Expected Outcomes Infant will have adequate metabolic function/be free of signs/symptoms of hyperbilirubinemia as evidenced by

a. total serum bilirubin level of less than 1.5 mg/100 ml
b. ability to tolerate feedings
c. pale yellow urine
d. yellow-brown stools
e. normal tone of cry
f. lack of

—jaundice
—extreme lethargy
—edema or ascites
—pruritus
—seizures

Possible Nursing Interventions

- Assess and record

  —infant's skin color and signs of itching every shift
  —signs of edema or ascites every 2 to 4 hours; measure abdominal girth if ordered and record results
  —any neurologic changes and vital signs every 2 hours
  —results of arterial blood gas analysis if ordered because acidosis causes increased levels of free unbound bilirubin and causes the albumin binding of bilirubin to weaken
  —Dextrostix as ordered; hypoglycemia will cause the breakdown of fats to yield free fatty acids that displace bilirubin from albumin
  —signs/symptoms of alteration in metabolic function/hyperbilirubinemia (such as those listed under "Characteristics") every 2 to 4 hours and PRN

- Assess and record bilirubin levels when they are ordered. Notify physician if levels are increasing.
- Keep infant unclothed under phototherapy lights with eyes covered. Remove infant from lights and remove eye pads for short periods so that nurse or parents can hold and comfort
- Keep accurate record of intake and output. Record characteristics of urine and stools. Anticipate increased fluid needs because of evaporative loss.
- Prevent chilling of infant to avoid raising levels of free fatty acids that displace bilirubin from its albumin binding sites.

- Prepare infant and family for exchange transfusion if indicated. Explain to the family the rationale for and specifics of the procedure. Follow hospital protocol for performing exchange transfusion. Monitor infant's vital signs continuously during exchange transfusion.

Evalution for Charting

- Describe infant's color.
- State highest and losest bilirubin levels.
- State whether phototherapy was used and whether infant was kept under lights unclothed and with eye pads.
- Describe any signs/symptoms of alteration in metabolic function/hyperbilirubinemia (such as those listed under "Characteristics").
- State abdominal girth and determine whether it has increased or decreased from previous measurement.
- State intake and output and characteristics of urine and stool.
- State range of vital signs and describe neurological status.
- State highest and lowest arterial pH values if ordered.
- State highest and lowest Dextrostix values if ordered.
- State whether an exchange transfusion was necessary and describe the infant's tolerance for the procedure.

ALTERATION IN LEVEL OF CONSCIOUSNESS

Nursing Diagnosis

Definition Reduced or impaired state of awareness; can range from mild to complete impairment

Possibly Related to   Deposition of unconjugated bilirubin in the brain cells

Characteristics   Lethargy
Seizures
High-pitched cry
Decrease in muscle tone
Opisthotonos

Expected Outcomes   Infant will maintain an appropriate level of consciousness as evidenced by

  a. being alert when awake
  b. normal-pitched cry
  c. muscle tone appropriate for gestational age
  d. lack of

    —seizures
    —opisthotonos

Possible Nursing Interventions

- Assess and record every 2 hours and PRN

  —alertness
  —cry
  —muscle tone
  —signs/symptoms of alteration in level of consciousness (such as those listed under "Characteristics")

- Reduce excessive stressors such as excessive handling, bright lights, and noise.
- Organize nursing care to minimize disturbance and stimulation of infant.

Evaluation for Charting

- Describe state of alertness, cry, and muscle tone.
- Describe any signs/symptoms of alteration in level of consciousness (such as those listed under "Characteristics").

- Describe any therapeutic measures used to minimize alerations in level of consciousness.

Related Nursing Diagnoses

ALTERATION IN NUTRITION: LESS THAN BODY REQUIREMENTS related to poor sucking and lethargy

DECREASED CARDIAC OUTPUT related to hemorrhage and polycythemia

IMPAIRED SKIN INTEGRITY related to pruritus and drying of skin due to phototherapy

INEFFECTIVE FAMILY COPING related to

a. incresed length of hospital stay
b. discoloration or infant's skin

Medical Diagnosis

HYPOCALCEMIA

Pathophysiology

Hypocalcemia is present when there is a serum calcium level of less than 7.0 mg/100 ml. Calcium metabolism is regulated in the body by the levels of intake, intestinal absorption, renal excretion, parathormone action, calcitonin levels, and amount of vitamin D present. In utero calcium is transported via the umbilical cord to the fetus. An interruption of this rapid calcium supply occurs at birth. Infants (even premature infants) have calcium reserves built up a birth, but calcium mobilization may be a problem. Parathyroid hormone activity is rarely detectable during the first few days of life, indicating decreased calcium mobilization. Vitamin D is needed for effective parathormone activity and may be inadequate in infants born during the winter and early spring. Calcitonin inhibits calcium mobilization, and the levels of calcitonin are generally increased in infants. Calcitonin levels are further increased by asphyxia.

Many factors predispose to hypocalcemia. These include maternal diabetes, maternal hyperparathyroidism, neonatal asphyxia, hypoxia, sepsis, and the administration of citrated blood. Left untreated, hypocalcemia can result in cardiac and respiratory arrest.

Primary Nursing Diagnosis

ALTERATION IN METABOLIC FUNCTION

Definition

Imbalance in the body's utilization of specific biochemicals

Possibly Related to
- Decreased levels of intake
- Decreased intestinal absorption
- Decreased renal excretion
- Decreased parathyroid hormone activity
- Increased calcitonin levels secondary to asphyxia
- Decreased amounts of vitamin D

Characteristics
Jitteriness
Irritability
Seizures
High-pitched cry
Cyanosis
Feeding difficulties
Chvostek's sign (tapping over the parotid gland causes spasms of facial muscles)
Trousseau's sign (pressing the principal vessels and nerves of a limb—B/P cuff inflated above systolic B/P for 3 minutes—produces spasmodic muscular contractions)

Expected Outcomes
Infant will have adequate metabolic function/lack of signs/symptoms of hypocalcemia as evidenced by

  a. total serum calcium level of 7.0 to 12.0 mg/100 ml
  b. ability to tolerate feedings
  c. normal tone of cry
  d. negative Chvostek's and Trousseau's signs
  e. lack of

  —jitteriness
  —extreme irritability
  —seizures

Possible Nursing Interventions
- Assess and record

—serum calcium levels as ordered. Notify physician if values are out of the stated range.

—signs/symptoms of hypocalcemia (such as those listed under "Characteristics") every 2 hours and PRN

- Keep accurate record of intake and output.
- Ensure that calcium is administered on schedule. It should be administered slowly by the IV route and the infant should be on a cardiac monitor. Rapid infusion can cause bradycardia and arrhythmias. Extravasation of calcium can lead to severe tissue necrosis. Calcium administered through an umbilical vein catheter that reaches the inferior vena cava can cause liver necrosis. Assess and record any side effects or complications.

Evaluation for Charting

- State highest and lowest serum calcium levels.
- Describe any signs/symptoms of hypocalcemia (such as those listed under "Characteristics").
- State intake and output.
- State whether calcium was administered on schedule and describe any side effects or complications.

ALTERATION IN LEVEL OF CONSCIOUSNESS

Nursing Diagnosis

Definition Reduced or impaired state of awareness; can range from mild to complete impairment

Possibly Related to Alteration in neuromuscular functioning

Characteristics Hyperalertness
Jitteriness
Irritability
High-pitched cry

Expected Outcomes Infant will maintain an appropriate level of consciousness as evidenced by

a. being appropriately alert when awake
b. normal-pitched cry
c. lack of
—jitteriness
—extreme irritability

Possible Nursing Interventions

- Assess and record every 2 hours and PRN

—alertness

—cry

—signs/symptoms of alteration in level of consciousness (such as those listed under "Characteristics")

- Reduce excessive stressors such as excessive handling, bright lights, and noise.
- Organize nursing care to minimize disturbance and stimulation of infant.

Evaluation for Charting

- Describe state of alertness and cry.
- Describe any signs/symptoms of alteration in level of consciousness (such as those listed under "Characteristics").
- Describe any therapeutic measures used to minimize alterations in level of consciousness.

Related Nursing Diagnoses DECREASED CARDIAC OUTPUT related to decreased myocardial contractility

ALTERATION IN NUTRITION: LESS THAN BODY REQUIREMENTS related to feeding difficulties

IMPAIRED SKIN INTEGRITY related to extravasation of IV calcium

INEFFECTIVE FAMILY COPING related to

a. increased length of hospital stay
b. invasive procedures (IV)

Medical Diagnosis	# HYPOGLYCEMIA

Pathophysiology Hypoglycemia can be defined as blood glucose levels of less than 40 mg/dl in term infants and of less than 30 mg/dl in premature infants. Low levels of blood glucose can be life-threatening for infants. Hypoglycemia may result in neurological impairment by producing cerebral swelling. In the premature infant, hypoglycemia occurs as a result of underdeveloped glycogen stores or inadequate caloric intake. Term infants may have depletion of glycogen stores due to stress secondary to a difficult delivery.

Primary Nursing Diagnosis ## ALTERATION IN METABOLIC FUNCTION

Definition Imbalance in the body's utilization of specific biochemicals

Possibly Related to
- Limited ability to mobilize glycogen stores
- Increased utilization of glucose due to physiologic stress

Characteristics Jitteriness, tremors
Apnea
Irregular respirations
Tachypnea
Cyanosis or grey color
Tachycardia
Lethargy
Irritability
Seizures
Feeding difficulties
Decrease in muscle tone
Hypothermia

Expected Outcomes Infant will have adequate metabolic function as evidenced by

    a. Dextrostix reading above 45 and below 160
    b. blood glucose level of 40 (30 in preterm infants) to 100 mg/dl
    c. regular respiratory rate within acceptable range of 30 to 60 breaths/minute
    d. heart rate within acceptable range of 100 to 160 beats/minute
    e. axillary temperature of 36.5° to 37.2° C
    f. muscle tone appropriate for gestational age
    g. lack of

        —cyanosis or grey color
        —lethargy
        —extreme irritability
        —seizures
        —feeding difficulties

Possible Nursing Interventions

- Assess and record

    —Dextrostix and serum glucose levels as ordered. Notify physician if values are out of the stated range.
    —vital signs every 2 hours and PRN
    —signs/symptoms of hypoglycemia (such as those listed under "Characteristics") every 2 hours and PRN

- Keep accurate record of intake and output.
- Administer and record glucose as ordered, either PO or IV. Assess and record effectiveness.

Evaluation for Charting	• State highest and lowest Dextrostix and blood glucose levels.
	• State highest and lowest range of vital signs.
	• Describe any signs/symptoms of hypoglycemia (such as those listed under "Characteristics").
	• State intake and output.
	• Describe any therapeutic measures used to prevent/correct hypoglycemia.

ALTERATION IN LEVEL OF CONSCIOUSNESS

Nursing Diagnosis

Definition

Reduced or impaired state of awareness; can range from mild to complete impairment

Possibly Related to

Lack of glucose for the central nervous system

Characteristics

Lethargy
Irritability
Seizures
High-pitched, weak cry
Decrease in muscle tone

Expected Outcomes

Infant will maintain an appropriate level of consciousness as evidenced by

    a. alertness when awake
    b. normal-pitched, strong cry
    c. muscle tone appropriate for gestational age
    d. lack of

       —lethargy
       —extreme irritability
       —seizures

Possible Nursing Interventions

• Assess and record every 2 hours and PRN

—alertness

—cry

—muscle tone

—signs/symptoms of alteration in level of consciousness (such as those listed under "Characteristics")

- Reduce excessive stressors such as handling, bright lights, and noise.
- Organize nursing care to minimize disturbance and stimulation of infant.

Evaluation for Charting

- Describe state of alertness, cry, and muscle tone.
- Describe any signs/symptoms of alteration in level of consciousness (such as those listed under "Characteristics").
- Describe any therapeutic measures used to minimize alterations in level of consciousness.

Related Nursing Diagnoses

IMPAIRED GAS EXCHANGE related to decreased oxygen consumption

ALTERNATION IN NUTRITION: LESS THAN BODY REQUIREMENTS related to insufficient amount of glucose in the blood

DECREASED CARDIAC OUTPUT related to poor cardiac contractility

INEFFECTIVE FAMILY COPING related to

a. increased length of hospital stay for infant

b. additional invasive procedures

INFANT OF DIABETIC MOTHER

Pathophysiology

Infants born of diabetic mothers (IDM) have a reported mortality rate of 15 to 25% when special care facilities are available. The mortality rate is affected by the length of gestation and the severity of the maternal diabetes. In addition, women with diabetes may also have other complications of pregnancy such as pregnancy-induced hypertension. The ideal delivery time for infants born of diabetic mothers is usually 36 to 38 weeks gestation. Term deliveries have been associated with a higher incidence of stillborn infants (probably due to placental insufficiency). Infants born of mothers not in good control are generally oversized for their gestational age, bloated, and flushed. Even though these infants appear large, they are still considered premature. They are oversized probably because of a sustained state of hyperglycemia (from high maternal blood sugars), which results in hyperinsulinism. These infants have hypertrophy and hyperplasia of the pancreatic islet cells from producing increased amounts of insulin, and this leads to excessive growth and deposition of fat.

Shortly after birth (usually within 2 to 4 hours), these infants become hypoglycemic because of the abrupt interruption of the maternal glucose supply. This decreased glucose supply along with increased amounts if insulin quickly depletes the blood of circulating glucose. Approximately 50% of these infants recover without complications.

Possible complications incude poly-cythemia, hyperbilirubinemia, and res-piratory distress syndrome. Infants born to mothers not in good control have a higher incidence of congenital anomalies such as cleft lip/palate and cardiac problems.

Primary Nursing Diagnosis

ALTERATION IN METABOLIC FUNCTION

Definition

Imbalance in the body's utilization of specific biochemicals

Possibly Related to

- Abrupt interruption of maternal glu-cose supply
- Hyperinsulinism
- Rebound hypoglycemia

Characteristics

Jitteriness, tremors
Apnea
Irregular respirations
Tachypnea
Cyanosis or grey color
Tachycardia
Lethargy
Irritability
Seizures
Feeding difficulties
Decrease in muscle tone
Hypothermia

Expected Outcomes

Infant will have adequate metabolic function/lack of signs/symptoms of hy-poglycemia as evicenced by

a. Dextrostix reading above 45 and below 160
b. blood glucose level between 40 (30 in preterm infants) and 100 mg/dl
c. regular respiratory rate within ac-ceptable range of 30 to 60 breaths/ minute

d. heart rate within acceptable range of 100 to 160 beats/minute
e. axillary temperature of 36.5° to 37.2° C
f. muscle tone appropriate for gestational age
g. lack of

—cyanosis or grey color
—lethargy
—extreme irritability
—seizures
—feeding difficulties

Possible Nursing Interventions

• Assess and record

—Dextrostix and serum glucose levels as ordered. Notify physician if values are out of the stated range.
—vital signs every 2 hours and PRN
—signs/symptoms of hypoglycemia (such as those listed under "Characteristics") every 2 hours and PRN

• Keep accurate record of intake and output.

• Administer and record glucose as ordered, either PO or IV. Early feedings of 5 to 10% glucose are usually recommended. Be aware that administration of glucose may trigger massive insulin release and rebound hypoglycemia. Assess and record effectiveness.

• Ensure that IM epinephrine (adrenaline) 1:10,000 is administered on schedule if ordered. It inhibits insulin release and stimulates release of glucose from glycogen stores. Assess and record any side effects (such as tachycardia and nausea).

Evaluation for Charting
- State highest and lowest Dextrostix and blood glucose levels.
- State highest and lowest range of vital signs.
- Describe any signs/symptoms of hypoglycemia (such as those listed under "Characteristics").
- State intake and output.
- Describe any therapeutic measures used to prevent/correct hypoglycemia.
- State whether epinephrine (adrenaline) was administered on schedule and describe any side effects.

ALTERATION IN LEVEL OF CONSCIOUSNESS

Nursing Diagnosis

Definition
Reduced or impaired state of awareness; can range from mild to complete impairment

Possibly Related to
Lack of glucose for the central nervous system

Characteristics
Lethargy
Irritability
Seizures
High-pitched, weak cry
Decrease in muscle tone

Expected Outcomes
Infant will maintain an appropriate level of consciousness as evidenced by

    a. alertness when awake
    b. normal-pitched, strong cry
    c. muscle tone appropriate for gestational age
    d. lack of

        —lethargy
        —extreme irritability
        —seizures

Possible Nursing Interventions

- Assess and record every 2 hours and PRN
  —alertness
  —cry
  —muscle tone
  —signs/symptoms of alteration in level of consciousness (such as those listed under "Characteristics")
- Reduce excessive stressors such as excessive handling, bright lights, and noise.
- Organize nursing care to minimize disturbance and stimulation of infant.

Evaluation for Charting

- Describe state of alertness, cry, and muscle tone.
- Describe any signs/symptoms of alteration in level of consciousness (such as those listed under "Characteristics").
- Describe any therapeutic measures used to minimize alterations in level of consciousness.

Related Nursing Diagnoses

IMPAIRED GAS EXCHANGE related to early delivery and prematurity

ALTERNATION IN NUTRITION: LESS THAN BODY REQUIREMENTS related to insufficient amount of glucose in the blood

DECREASED CARDIAC OUTPUT related to poor cardiac contractility

INEFFECTIVE FAMILY COPING related to

a. increased length of hospital stay for infant
b. additional invasive procedures
c. maternal guilt

Medical Diagnosis	# HYPERVISCOSITY/"THICK BLOOD" SYNDROME
Pathophysiology	Hyperviscosity or the "thick blood" syndrome occurs when there is sludging of blood, which can cause obstruction of small capillaries. It is associated with polycythemia, which is defined as a central hematocrit of 65% or greater. The obstruction of capillaries can lead to neurological, gastrointestinal, respiratory, and renal problems. There are many predisposing factors, including milking of the umbilical cord, chronic intrauterine hypoxia, intrauterine growth retardation, postmaturity, a diabetic mother, high altitudes, hypoxia, and chromosomal abnormalities. Hyperviscosity can lead to complications such as intraventricular hemorrhage, necrotizing enterocolitis, and renal vein thrombosis.
Primary Nursing Diagnosis	## ALTERATION IN TISSUE PERFUSION
Definition	Inadequate amount of blood and oxygen being delivered to the tissues in the body
Possibly Related to	Increased number of red blood cells secondary to • birth at high altitude • hypoxia • late cord clamping • milking of umbilical cord • holding infant down while cord still pulsating
Characteristics	Plethora Lethargy Decreased alertness Tremors Seizures

Decreased muscle tone
Weak suck
Cyanosis
Jaundice
Hepatomegaly
Chest x-ray revealing hyperaerated lungs and vascular engorgement

Expected Outcomes

Infant will have adequate tissue perfusion as evidenced by

a. hematocrit of 50 to 60%
b. alertness when awake
c. strong suck
d. clear chest x-ray
e. muscle tone appropriate for gestational age
f. lack of

—plethora
—seizures
—cyanosis
—jaundice
—hepatomegaly

Possible Nursing Interventions

- Assess and record

—hematocrit levels as ordered. Notify physician if values are out of the stated range.
—alertness, color, and muscle tone every 2 hours and PRN
—signs/symptoms of alteration in tissue perfusion (such as those listed under "Characteristics") every 2 hours and PRN

- Check and record results of chest x-ray when indicated.
- Prepare infant and family for exchange transfusion (plasma is used to replace blood) if indicated. Explain to the family the rationale for and specifics of the procedure. Follow hospi-

tal protocol for performing exchange transfusion. Monitor infant's vital signs continuously during exchange transfusion.

Evaluation for Charting

- State highest and lowest hematocrit levels.
- Describe infant's color, muscle tone, and state of alertness.
- Describe any signs/symptoms of alteration in tissue perfusion (such as those listed under "Characteristics").
- Describe results of chest x-ray if available.
- State whether an exchange transfusion was necessary and, if so, the infant's level of tolerance for procedure.

ALTERATION IN LEVEL OF CONSCIOUSNESS

Nursing Diagnosis

Definition Reduced or impaired state of awareness; can range from mild to complete impairment

Possibly Related to Characteristics
Decreased cerebral blood flow
Lethargy
Decreased alertness
Tremors
Seizures
Decreased muscle tone

Expected Outcomes
Infant will maintain an appropriate level of consciousness as evidenced by

a. alertness when awake
b. muscle tone appropriate for gestational age
c. lack of

—tremors
—seizures

Possible Nursing Interventions

- Assess and record every 2 hours and PRN
  —state of alertness
  —muscle tone
  —signs/symptoms of alteration in level of consciousness (such as those listed under "Characteristics")
- Reduce excessive stressors such as excessive handling, bright lights, and noise.
- Organize nursing care to minimize disturbance and stimulation of infant.

Evaluation for Charting

- Describe muscle tone and state of alertness.
- Describe any signs/symptoms of alteration in level of consciousness (such as those listed under "Characteristics").
- Describe any therapeutic measures used to minimize alteration in level of consciousness.

Related Nursing Diagnoses

IMPAIRED GAS EXCHANGE related to decreased pulmonary blood flow

DECREASED CARDIAC OUTPUT related to increased workload on the heart secondary to viscous blood

ALTERATION IN METABOLIC FUNCTION related to increased bilirubin levels secondary to increased number of red blood cells

INEFFECTIVE FAMILY COPING related to invasive procedures such as exchange transfusion

Medical Diagnosis	# SEPSIS

Pathophysiology

Sepsis is defined as a generalized bacterial invasion of the bloodstream. Normally, immunoglobulins are transferred from the mother and stored in fetal tissue during the final weeks of gestation. Premature infants have a lack of immunoglobulins due to the interruption of gestation. The immune system of the premature infant is immature, which causes reduced function of circulating white blood cells. This, along with hypofunction of the adrenal glands, allows rapid invasion, spread, and multiplication of organisms. The most frequent infectious agents are group B streptococci and *Staphylococcus epidermidis*. Before the advent of antibiotics, the mortality rate for infants with sepsis was 90%. It is now approximately 13 to 45%.

Primary Nursing Diagnosis

ACTUAL INFECTION

Definition

A condition in which the body is invaded by microorganisms

Possibly Related to

- Prolonged rupture of membranes
- Intrauterine infection
- Prolonged labor and fetel distress
- Obstetrical manipulation
- Maternal illness
- Congenital malformations
- Trauma
- Immature immune system
- Nosocomial source
- Unknown cause

Characteristics

General Signs
Infant generally "not doing well"
Temperature instability

Cardiovascular
Pallor, cyanosis, mottling
Cold, clammy skin
Hypotension
Edema
Bradycardia/tachycardia
Respiratory
Apnea
Tachypnea
Cyanosis
Grunting
Dyspnea
Retractions
Central Nervous System
Lethargy, hyporeflexia, coma
Irritability, tremors, seizures
Full fontanel
Increased or decreased tone
Gastrointestinal
Feeding difficulties
Vomiting
Diarrhea or decreased stool
Abdominal distention
Hepatomegaly
Hypoglycemia/hyperglycemia
Hematopoietic System
Jaundice
Pallor
Purpura, petechiae, ecchymosis
Splenomegaly
Bleeding
Neutropenia
Thrombocytopenia

Expected Outcomes

Infant will be free of infection as evidenced by

a. axillary temperature between 36.5° and 37.2° C
b. regular respiratory rate within acceptable range of 30 to 60 breaths/minute

c. heart rate within acceptable range of 100 to 160 beats/minute
d. B/P within acceptable range of 64/30 to 96/62 mm Hg
e. blood glucose between 40 (30 in preterm infants) and 100 mg/dl
f. white blood cell count within normal limits of 9,000 to 30,000 mm^3
g. platelet count within normal limits of 100,000 to 400,000 mm^3
h. lack of signs/symptoms of infection (such as those listed under "Characteristics")

Possible Nursing Interventions

- Assess and record every 2 hours and PRN

  —vital signs
  —signs/symptoms of infection (such as those listed under "Characteristics")

- Maintain a neutral thermal environment.
- Ensure that antibiotics are given on schedule. Assess and record any side effects (such as rash or diarrhea).
- Assess IV site every hour for signs/symptoms of infection or infiltration. Record findings at least once/shift.
- Use sterile technique when doing procedures such as suctioning and changing IV tubing.
- Maintain good handwashing technique, especially between patients.
- Assess parents'/visitors' knowledge of handwashing technique; correct as needed.
- Maintain isolation if indicated.
- Check and record results of laboratory work such as blood cultures and CBC.

Evaluation for Charting
- State highest and lowest range of vital signs.
- Describe any signs/symptoms of infection (such as those listed under "Characteristics").
- Describe whether a neutral thermal environment was maintained.
- State whether antibiotics were administered on schedule and describe any side effects.
- Describe IV site.
- State whether parents/visitors demonstrated correct handwashing technique?
- If isolation was necessary, describe type needed.
- State laboratory results if available.

Nursing Diagnosis

INEFFECTIVE BREATHING PATTERN

Definition
A breathing pattern that results in oxygen insufficient to meet the cellular requirements of the body

Possibly Related to
- Tachypnea
- Periodic breathing/apnea

Characteristics
Tachypnea
Apnea
Cyanosis
Grunting
Dyspnea
Retractions

Expected Outcomes
Infant will maintain effective breathing as evidenced by

  a. respiratory rate within the acceptable range of 30 to 60 breaths/minute
  b. clear and equal breath sounds
  c. lack of

    —cyanosis

—grunting
—retractions

Possible Nursing Interventions

- Assess and record every 2 hours and PRN

    —respiratory rate and breath sounds
    —signs/symptoms of ineffective breathing pattern (such as those listed under "Characteristics")

- Ensure that oxygen is being delivered in the correct amount and by the correct route. Record percentage of liter flow and route of delivery every 2 hours. State effectiveness of treatment.
- If intubated, check ventilator settings (FiO2, Rate, PIP, TV, PEEP/CPAP) every 15 minutes. Record every 1 to 2 hours. Suction endotracheal tube using sterile technique every 2 to 3 hours and PRN. Record amount and characteristics of secretions.
- Reposition infant every 2 hours unless contraindicated.

Evaluation for Charting

- State highest and lowest respiratory rate.
- Describe breath sounds.
- Describe any signs/symptoms of an ineffective breathing pattern (such as those listed under "Characteristics").
- State amount, route, and effectiveness of oxygen therapy.
- State type of endotracheal tube in place and ventilator settings.
- Describe amount and characteristics of secretions.
- State whether infant was repositioned every 2 hours?

Related Nursing Diagnoses

FLUID VOLUME DEFICIT related to

  a. ineffective thermoregulation
  b. decreased appetite
  c. side effects of antibiotics

DECREASED CARDIAC OUTPUT related to

  a. abnormal heart beat
  b. decreased blood pressure
  c. bleeding

ALTERATION IN LEVEL OF CONSCIOUSNESS related to altered activity level

INEFFECTIVE FAMILY COPING related to

  a. illness of infant
  b. prolonged hospital stay
  c. possible complication of disease state

**Section 2
Pediatric Critical Care Plans**

Medical Diagnosis	# BACTERIAL MENINGITIS

Pathophysiology

Meningitis is defined as inflammation of the meninges (the protective membrane covering the brain and spinal cord). Bacterial meningitis results when the meninges are invaded by bacteria via the bloodstream from various possible foci of infection. Organisms can also directly invade the meninges after head trauma, penetrating wounds, and neurosurgical procedures. As a result of this invasion, inflammation occurs. Accordingly, there is an increase in the white blood cell count, an exudate forms, cerebrospinal fluid secretion increases, and the brain becomes hyperemic and edematous. *Haemophilus influenzae* (type B), *Neisseria meningitidis* (meningococcus), and *Streptococcus pneumoniae* are the bacterial organisms most likely to cause meningitis in children.

Primary Nursing Diagnosis

ALTERATION IN LEVEL OF CONSCIOUSNESS

Definition

Reduced or impaired state of awareness; can range from mild to complete impairment (coma)

Possibly Related to

An inflammation of the meninges (state specific organism if known)

Characteristics

Fever
Headache
Irritability
Lethargy
Vomiting
Poor feeding
Bulging fontanel
Nuchal rigidity

Change in level of consciousness
High-pitched cry
Pupillary changes
Positive Kernig and Brudzinski signs
Seizures
Apnea
Increase in head circumference

Expected Outcomes

Child will maintain an appropriate level of consciousness as evidenced by

a. pupils that are equal and react to light
b. equal movement of all extremities
c. normal-pitched cry
d. age-appropriate reflexes
e. age-appropriate response to pain
f. being alert when awake
g. oriented × 3 (if age-appropriate)
h. recognition of family members (if age-appropriate)
i. lack of lethargy

Child will be free of signs/symptoms of increased intracranial pressure as evidenced by

a. spontaneous respirations within acceptable range (state specific highest and lowest rates for each child)
b. heart rate within acceptable range (state specific highest and lowest rates for each child)
c. pulse pressure within acceptable limits of 20 to 50 mm Hg
d. systolic pressure within acceptable range (state specific highest and lowest systolic pressures for each child)
e. temperature within acceptable range of 35.6° to 37.2° C

f. lack of signs/symptoms listed under "Characteristics"

- Assess and record the following every 1 to 2 hours and PRN

  —neurological vital signs (use Glasgow Coma Scale if available)
  —vital signs
  —signs/symptoms of increased intracranial pressure (such as those listed under "Characteristics")
  —signs/symptoms of decreasing level of consciousness (such as those listed under "Characteristics")

- Measure and record head circumference daily.
- Elevate head of bed at a 30° angle.
- Keep acurate record of intake and output.
- Restrict fluid intake as ordered (usually 1/2 to 2/3 maintenance).
- Maintain child's body temperature between 35.6° and 37.2° C.
- Keep environment as quiet as possible.
- Organize nursing care to minimize disturbance and stimulation of the child.
- Ensure that antibiotics, antipyretics, and anticonvulsants are administered on schedule. Assess and record effectiveness and any side effects (such as diarrhea, rash, vomiting, and sedation).

**Evaluation
for Charting**

- State range of vital signs.
- Describe neurologic signs.
- Describe any signs/symptoms of increased intracranial pressure and de-

creasing level of consciousness (such as those listed under "Characteristics").
- Describe any therapeutic measures used to decrease intracranial pressure and their effectiveness.
- State intake and output.
- State whether medications were administered on schedule and describe any side effects.

Nursing Diagnosis   **ALTERATION IN COMFORT**

Definition   A condition in which an individual experiences discomfort

Possibly Related to
- Headache
- Neck pain
- Earache
- Fever
- Procedures/treatments

Characteristics   Verbal communication of discomfort

Constant crying unrelieved by usual comfort measures

Facial grimacing

Physical signs/symptoms
     Tachycardia
     Tachypnea/bradypnea
     Increased blood pressure
     Diaphoresis
     Pupillary dilation

Expected Outcomes   Child will be free of severe/constant discomfort as evidenced by

     a. verbal communication of comfort
     b. lack of constant crying
     c. lack of facial expression of discomfort
     d. heart rate within acceptable range (state specific highest and lowest rates for each child)

e. respiratory rate within acceptable range (state specific highest and lowest rates for each child)
f. blood pressure within acceptable range (state specific highest and lowest pressures for each child)
g. lack of

—diaphoresis
—dilated pupils

Possible Nursing Interventions

- Assess and record any signs/symptoms of discomfort (such as those listed under "Characteristics") at least once/shift.
- Handle child gently.
- Encourage family members to stay and comfort child when possible.
- Allow family members to participate in the care of the child when possible.
- Use distraction measures (listening to music box) when appropriate.
- Ensure that antipyretics and antibiotics are administered on schedule. Assess for effectiveness and any side effects (such as rash, diarrhea).

Evaluation for Charting

- State range of vital signs.
- Describe any signs/symptoms of discomfort.
- Describe any successful measures used to reduce discomfort.
- If antipyretics were given, describe effectiveness.
- Describe effectiveness of antibiotics and any side effects.

Related Nursing Diagnoses

FLUID VOLUME DEFICIT related to

a. poor feeding

b. vomiting

c. fever

INEFFECTIVE THERMOREGULA-
TION related to the infection of the
meninges

DEVELOPMENTAL DELAY related
to

a. possible brain damage secondary
to increased intracranial pressure

b. cerebral infarcts

c. brain abscesses

INEFFECTIVE FAMILY COPING
related to hospitalization of child
with a serious illness

Medical Diagnosis	# ENCEPHALITIS

Pathophysiology

Encephalitis is an inflammation of the brain parenchyma. The inflammation occurs when the brain is directly invaded by an infectious pathogen, most frequently a virus. Pathologic changes in the brain may include edema, cellular damage, petechial hemorrhages, necrosis, the appearance of inclusion bodies, neuronal degeneration, and demyelination.

Primary Nursing Diagnosis

ALTERATION IN LEVEL OF CONSCIOUSNESS

Definition

Reduced or impaired state of awareness; can range from mild to complete impairment (coma)

Possibly Related to

An inflammation of brain parenchyma secondary to a pathogenic invasion (usually viral)

Characteristics

Malaise
Fever
Headache
Dizziness
Apathy
Nuchal rigidity
Nausea
Vomiting
Ataxia
Tremors
Hyperactivity
Visual, auditory, and/or speech disturbances
Seizures
Aphasia, sudden onset
Hemiplegia, sudden onset
Behavioral changes

Expected Outcomes

Child will maintain an appropriate level of consciousness as evidenced by

  a. pupils that are equal and react to light
  b. normal-pitched cry
  c. equal movement of all extremities
  d. age-appropriate reflexes
  e. age-appropriate response to pain
  f. being alert when awake
  g. oriented ×3 (if age-appropriate)
  h. recognition of family members (if age-appropriate)
  i. age-appropriate developmental level (state individualized examples for each child)
  j. ability to perform age-appropriate activities of daily living (state individualized examples for each child)
  k. lack of lethargy

Child will be free of signs/symptoms of increased intracranial pressure as evidenced by

  a. spontaneous respirations within acceptable range (state specific highest and lowest rates for each child)
  b. heart rate within acceptable range (state specific highest and lowest rates for each child)
  c. pulse pressure within acceptable limits of 20 to 50 mm Hg
  d. systolic pressure within acceptable range (state specific highest and lowest systolic pressures for each child)
  e. temperature within acceptable range of 35.6° to 37.2° C

Possible Nursing Interventions

f. lack of signs/symptoms listed under "Characteristics"

- Assess and record the following every 1 to 2 hours and PRN

  —neurologic vital signs (use Glasgow Coma Scale if available)
  —vital signs
  —signs/symptoms of increased intracranial pressure (such as those listed under "Characteristics")

- Keep accurate record of intake and output.
- Restrict fluid intake as ordered (usually 1/2 to 2/3 maintenance).
- Elevate head of bed at a 30° angle; maintain head in midline position.
- Maintain child's body temperature between 35.6° and 37.2° C.
- Keep environment as quiet as possible.
- Organize nursing care to minimize disturbance and stimulation of the child.
- Ensure that antibiotics/antiviral agents, antipyretics, and anticonvulsants are administered on schedule. Assess and record effectiveness and any side effects (such as diarrhea, rash, vomiting, and sedation).

Evaluation for Charting

- State range of vital signs.
- Describe neurologic signs.
- Describe signs/symptoms of increased intracranial pressure (such as those under "Characteristics").
- Describe any therapeutic measures used to decrease intracranial pressure and their effectiveness.
- State intake and output.

- State whether medications were administered on schedule? Describe any side effects.

Nursing Diagnosis | **INEFFECTIVE BREATHING PATTERN**

Definition | A breathing pattern that results in oxygen insufficient to meet the cellular requirements of the body

Possibly Related to | Increased intracranial pressure secondary to cerebral edema
Pain
Immobility

Characteristics | Tachypnea or bradypnea, apnea
Irritability
Restlessness
Diminished breath sounds
Fever
Retractions
Nasal flaring
Bradycardia

Expected Outcomes | Child will have an effective breathing pattern as evidenced by

    a. respiratory rate within acceptable range (state specific high and low rates for each child)
    b. clear and equal breath sounds bilaterally
    c. lack of retractions and nasal flaring
    d. body temperature maintained between 36.5° and 37.2° C

Possible Nursing Interventions | • Assess and record every 1 to 2 hours and PRN

    —breath sounds with vital signs
    —signs/symptoms of ineffective breathing pattern (such as those listed under "Characteristics").

- Assess effectiveness of oxygen therapy, if ordered. Record percentage of liter flow and route of delivery.
- Ensure that antipyretics are administered as indicated. Assess and record for effectiveness.
- Position child so that airway is in neutral (sniff) position.
- Elevate head of bed at a 30° angle unless contraindicated.

Evaluation for Charting

- State highest and lowest respiratory rates.
- Describe breath sounds.
- Describe any signs/symptoms of ineffective breathing pattern (such as those listed under "Characteristics").
- Chart whether oxygen therapy was administered and state amount and route of delivery. Describe effectiveness of treatment.

Related Nursing Diagnosis

ALTERATION IN COMFORT: PAIN related to brain irritation/inflammation secondary to pathogenic invasion.

IMPAIRMENT OF SKIN INTEGRITY related to

a. immobility
b. dehydration
c. diaphoresis

POTENTIAL FOR FURTHER INFECTION related to invasive procedures

ALTERATION IN FAMILY COPING related to critical nature of the situation and uncertain prognosis

Medical Diagnosis	# GUILLAIN-BARRÉ SYNDROME
Pathophysiology	Guillain Barré Syndrome (GBS) is a progressive polyneuritis (inflammation of many nerves) of unknown cause. There is decreased speed and intensity of peripheral and/or cranial nerve conduction as the myelin sheath is destroyed and demyelinization occurs. GBS is characterized by a prickling sensation in the hands and feet and pain, with eventual paralysis. Symmetrical motor weakness begins in the lower extremities and advances rapidly upward. GBS is usually preceded by an upper respiratory infection or viral illness, which appears 2 to 3 weeks before the onset of GBS. Approximately 4 to 8 weeks after the appearance of symptoms, recovery begins. In the pediatric age group GBS most commonly occurs in children 4 to 10 years of age.
Primary Nursing Diagnosis	## INEFFECTIVE AIRWAY CLEARANCE
Definition	Inability to clear secretions from the airways adequately
Possibly Related to	Neuromuscular dysfunction of the facial, throat, and respiratory muscles
Characteristics	Change in respiratory rate, shallow irregular respirations Diminished breath sounds Difficulty swallowing Pooling of secretions Pallor, cyanosis Decreased chest expansion Breathlessness in vocalizations Tachypnea, dyspnea Hypercarbia

Expected Outcomes

Child will have adequate airway clearance as evidenced by

    a. respiratory rate within acceptable range (state specific highest and lowest rates for each child)
    b. clear and equal breath sounds bilaterally
    c. lack of cyanosis
    d. adequate chest expansion
    e. ability to clear secretions by coughing
    f. clear audible vocalizations
    g. ability to swallow secretions

Possible Nursing Interventions

- Assess and record every 1 to 2 hours and PRN

    —respiratory rate and breath sounds
    —any signs/symptoms of ineffective airway clearance (such as those listed under "Characteristics")
    —amount and characteristics of secretions
    —ability to cough and swallow
    —status of speech
    —arterial blood gas results. Notify physician of any abnormalities.

- Assist child with coughing and deep breathing, i.e., use of bedside spirometer.
- Provide gentle nasotracheal and oropharyngeal suctioning as needed.
- Administer oxygen as ordered, record percentage of liter flow and route of delivery. Assess for effectiveness every 2 hours.
- If child is intubated

    —check ventilator settings (FiO2, Rate, PIP or TV, PEEP/CPAP) ev-

ery 15 minutes. Record every 1 to 2 hours.
—suction using sterile technique every 2 hours and PRN.

- Ensure that chest physiotherapy is being done effectively and on schedule.
- Elevate head of bed at a 30° angle, unless contraindicated.

Evaluation for Charting

- State highest and lowest respiratory rates.
- Describe breath sounds.
- Describe any signs/symptoms of ineffective airway clearance (such as those listed under "Characteristics").
- State frequency of suctioning and describe characteristics of secretions.
- State highest and lowest arterial blood gas values and state the ongoing physiological process (i.e., respiratory acidosis).
- State type of endotracheal tube used and ventilator settings.
- Describe child's response to chest physiotherapy.
- State whether head of bed was elevated at a 30° angle?

Nursing Diagnosis

DECREASED CARDIAC OUTPUT

Definition

A decrease in the amount of blood that leaves the left ventricle

Possibly Related to Characteristics

Autonomic dysfunction
Dysrhythmias
Tachycardia
Bradycardia
Cyanosis
Episodic diaphoresis
Dizziness

Pallor of skin and mucous membranes, flushed face
Oliguria, anuria
Labile blood pressure
Weak peripheral pulses
Prolonged capillary refill, longer than 2 to 3 seconds

Expected Outcomes

Child will maintain an adequate cardiac output as evidenced by

a. heart rate within acceptable range (state specific highest and lowest rates for each child)
b. blood pressure within acceptable range (state specific highest and lowest blood pressures for each child)
c. normal sinus rhythm
d. strong and equal peripheral pulses
e. brisk capillary refill, within 2 to 3 seconds
f. skin warm to touch
g. pink and moist mucous membranes
h. adequate urine output (state specific highest and lowest outputs for each child; normal, 1 to 2 ml/kg/hour)
i. lack of

—cyanosis
—dizziness

Possible Nursing Interventions

• Access and record every 2 to 4 hours and PRN

—apical rate and blood pressure
—any signs/symptoms of decreased cardiac output (such as those listed under "Characteristics")

- Evaluate and record results of EKG strips at least once/shift.
- Keep accurate record of intake and output.
- Administer cardiac drugs (digoxin, atropine sulfate, and/or hydralazine hydrochloride) on schedule if ordered. Assess and record effectiveness.
- Administer volume expanders or colloid solutions on schedule if ordered. Assess and record effectiveness.

Evaluation for Charting

- State highest and lowest apical rates and B/P.
- Describe any signs/symptoms of decreased cardiac output (such as those listed under "Characteristics").
- Document EKG interpretation.
- State intake and output.
- Describe any therapeutic measures used to increase cardiac output and their effectiveness.

Nursing Diagnosis   **IMPAIRED PHYSICAL MOBILITY**

Definition   Limited ability of movement

Possibly Related to

- Pain
- Weakness
- Paralysis secondary to demyelinization

Characteristics   Inability to move part or all of the body

Decreased range of motion

Limited or decreased coordination

Paraparesis

Quadriplegia

Complete areflexia

Paresthesias

Decreased muscle strength, control, or mass

Expected Outcomes

Child will return to preillness activity level before illness (state specific examples for each child)

Possible Nursing Interventions

- Assess and record child's activity level at least once/shift.
- Assess and record any signs/symptoms of impaired physical mobility (such as those listed under "Characteristics").
- Arrange for play therapy, occupational therapy, and/or physical therapy when appropriate.
- Encourage child to take an active role in own care.
- Encourage and make available activities that the child can do within own limitations.
- Allow adequate rest periods (state specific amount of rest needed for each child).
- Perform scheduled active and passive range of motion.
- Ensure that child's body stays in proper alignment.
- Turn child every 2 hours (or as indicated).
- Massage bony prominences every 4 to 8 hours to prevent skin breakdown.
- Use foot board/leg splints/high-top tennis shoes to prevent foot-drop.
- Use sheepskin and/or special beds for comfort and to prevent skin breakdown when indicated.

Evaluation for Charting

- Describe child's present level of activity.

- Describe any signs/symptoms of impaired physical mobility (such as those listed under "Characteristics").
- State child's ability to participate and/or limitations from participating in own care.
- Describe any therapeutic measures used to improve physical mobility and their effectiveness.

Related Nursing Diagnoses

IMPAIRED SKIN INTEGRITY related to

a. impaired physical mobility
b. prolonged bedrest
c. sensorimotor deficits

IMPAIRED VERBAL COMMUNICATION related to paralysis

FEAR, CHILD'S related to

a. loss of function
b. uncertain prognosis
c. procedures/treatments

Medical
Diagnosis

HEMATOMAS/VASCULAR HEAD INJURIES

Pathophysiology

One of the major complications of head trauma is hemorrhage due to a break in the wall of a blood vessel, usually resulting in a localized collection of blood.

With an epidural hematoma, blood accumulates between the skull and the dura mater. The bleeding most often is arterial, accumulating rapidly from a tear in the middle meningeal artery. An epidural hematoma is usually associated with a skull fracture caused by a low-velocity blow to the skull.

A subdural hematoma is an accumulation of blood between the dura mater and the arachnoid membranes. It usually results from rupture of the cortical veins that bridge the subdural space. Subdural hematomas are further classified as acute, subacute, or chronic. Collections of blood that occur within hours after a head injury are called acute subdural hematomas. A subacute subdural hematoma also occurs early, but after a less severe head injury; it produces increased intracranial pressure with loss of consciousness. Chronic subdural hematomas occur after minor head injuries; the blood accumulates slowly over weeks or months.

Severe head injuries may cause a subarachnoid hemorrhage, in which blood accumulates from torn subarachnoid vessels.

Primary Nursing Diagnosis	**ALTERATION IN LEVEL OF CONSCIOUSNESS**
Definition	Reduced or impaired state of awareness; can range from mild to complete impairment (coma)
Possibly Related to	Increased intracranial pressure secondary to blood accumulation between the skull and cerebral surfaces.
Characteristics	*Epidural*

Epidural
Decreased responsiveness
Initial lucid period
Unilateral pupil dilation (usually ipsilateral to the hemorrhage)
Change in level of consciousness
Contralateral weakness or paralysis
Increased deep tendon reflexes
Decerebrate activity
Headache
Nausea/vomiting
Drowsiness
Bradycardia

Subdural
Seizures
Vomiting
Irritability
Drowsiness
Personality changes
Headache
Unsteady gait
Apnea
Increased head circumference
Bulging fontanel
Retinal hemorrhages
Hemiparesis
Quadriplegia
Mild obtundation
Deep coma
Decerebrate posturing
Flaccidity

Subarachnoid
Seizures
Headache
Nuchal rigidity
Change in level of consciousness
Ipsilateral pupil dilation
Hemiparesis

**Expected
Outcomes**

Child will maintain an appropriate level of consciousness as evidenced by

a. pupils that are equal and react to light
b. equal movement of all extremities
c. flat fontanel
d. stable head circumference
e. normal-pitched cry
f. age-appropriate reflexes
g. age-appropriate response to pain
h. alertness when awake
i. orientation ×3 (if age-appropriate)
j. recognition of family members (if age-appropriate)
k. age-appropriate developmental level (state individualized examples for each child)
l. ability to perform age-appropriate activities of daily living (state individualized examples for each child)

Child will be free of signs/symptoms of increased intracranial pressure as evidenced by

a. spontaneous respirations within acceptable range (state specific highest and lowest rates for each child)
b. heart rate within acceptable range (state specific highest and lowest rates for each child)

c. pulse pressure within acceptable limits of 20 to 50 mm Hg
d. systolic pressure within acceptable range (state specific highest and lowest systolic pressures for each child)
e. lack of signs/symptoms listed under "Characteristics"

Possible Nursing Interventions

- Assess and record the following every 1 to 2 hours and PRN

  —neurologic vital signs (use Glasgow Coma scale if available)
  —vital signs
  —signs/symptoms of increased intracranial pressure (such as those listed under "Characteristics")
  —any drainage from ears, nose, or mouth

- Keep acurate record of intake and output.
- Elevate head of bed at a 30° angle (unless contraindicated).
- Maintain head in midline position.
- Keep environment as quiet as possible.
- Organize nursing care to minimize disturbance and stimulation of the child.
- Ensure that anticonvulsants, diuretics, steroids, antipyretics, and antibiotics are administered on schedule. Assess and record effectiveness and any side effects (such as nausea, vomiting, and rash).
- Prepare child for any invasive procedures and/or surgical treatments such as intracranial catheter placement and craniotomy.

Evaluation for Charting

- Explain to the child's family any indicated procedure and its rationale.
- State range of vital signs.
- Describe neurologic signs.
- Describe signs/symptoms of increased intracranial pressure (such as those listed under "Characteristics").
- Describe any therapeutic measures used to decrease intracranial pressure and their effectiveness.
- State intake and output.
- State whether medications were administered on schedule and describe any side effects.
- Describe child's level of tolerance for any invasive and/or surgical procedures that might have been done.
- If procedures were done, state whether child showed any signs of improvement after the procedure.

Nursing Diagnosis

INEFFECTIVE BREATHING PATTERN

Definition

A breathing pattern that results in oxygen insufficient to meet the cellular requirements of the body

Possibly Related to

- Increased intracranial pressure secondary to blood accumulation between the skull and cerebral surfaces
- Apnea
- Bradypnea/Tachypnea

Characteristics

Tachypnea/bradypnea
Apnea
Irritability
Restlessness
Drowsiness
Retractions
Nasal flaring

Expected Outcomes

Child will have an effective breathing pattern as evidenced by

    a. respiratory rate within acceptable range (state specific high and low rates for each child)

    b. clear and equal breath sounds bilaterally

    c. lack of retractions and nasal flaring

Possible Nursing Interventions

- Assess and record every 1 to 2 hours and PRN

    —breath sounds with vital signs

    —signs/symptoms of ineffective breathing pattern (such as those listed under "Characteristics").

- Assess effectiveness of oxygen therapy, if ordered. Record percentage of liter flow and route of delivery.
- Position child so that airway is in neutral (sniff) position.
- Elevate head of bed at a 30° angle unless contraindicated.

Evaluation for Charting

- State highest and lowest respiratory rate.
- Describe breath sounds.
- Describe any signs/symptoms of ineffective breathing pattern (such as those listed under "Characteristics").
- Chart whether oxygen therapy was administered and state amount and route of delivery. Describe effectiveness of treatment.

Related Nursing Diagnoses

DECREASED CARDIAC OUTPUT related to

    a. bradycardia/tachycardia secondary to increased intracranial pressure

    b. dysrhythmias secondary to increased intracranial pressure
    c. hemorrhage secondary to head trauma
    d. decreased oxygenation

ALTERATION IN NUTRITION: LESS THAN BODY REQUIREMENTS related to

    a. nausea/vomiting
    b. fatigue
    c. anorexia
    d. decreased level of consciousness
    e. difficulty swallowing or chewing
    f. loss of appetite

DEVELOPMENTAL DELAY related to sequelae of head trauma

CHILD'S FEAR related to

    a. disorientation
    b. hospital environment
    c. invasive procedures

Medical Diagnosis	# NEUROSURGERY, POSTOPERATIVE CARE

Pathophysiology

Neurosurgery may be required for the pediatric patient for a variety of reasons. These reasons include the correction, care, or repair of malformations or traumatic lesions of the nervous system, surgical treatment of diseases of the nervous system, and surgical palliation of pain. The goal of neurosurgery is to restore the child to his/her optimal level of neurologic functioning within the disease state.

The postoperative period is a critical time. The establishment of vital functions is of primary concern. Continual, thorough assessments must be performed to determine the degree of neurologic compromise and the adequacy of ventilation and systemic perfusion. Postoperative complications include increased intracranial pressure, seizures, the syndrome of inappropriate antidiuretic hormone, diabetes insipidus, and infection.

Primary Nursing Diagnosis

ALTERATION IN LEVEL OF CONSCIOUSNESS

Definition

Reduced or impaired state of awareness; can range from mild to complete impairment

Possibly Related to

- Increased intracranial pressure secondary to cerebral edema
- Increased intracranial pressure secondary to increased blood volume
- Increased intracranial pressure secondary to increased cerebrospinal fluid
- Seizures

Characteristics   Lethargy
Irritability
Vomiting
Anorexia
Poor feeding
Bulging fontanel
Headache
High-pitched cry
Blurred vision
Papilledema
Change in level of consciousness
Sluggish pupillary response to light
Unequal pupils
Tachycardia
Bradycardia
Systolic hypertension
Widened pulse pressure
Apnea
Decorticate rigidity or decerebrate posturing
Absence of gag or cough
Increased head circumference

Expected Outcomes   Child will maintain an appropriate level of consciousness as evidenced by

    a. pupils that are equal and react to light
    b. equal movement of all extremities
    c. age-appropriate reflexes
    d. age-appropriate response to pain
    e. alertness when awake
    f. orientation X3 (if age-appropriate)
    g. recognition of family members (if age-appropriate)
    h. age-appropriate developmental level (state individualized examples for each child)
    i. ability to perform age-appropriate activities of daily living (state indvidualized examples for each child)

Child will be free of signs/symptoms of increased intracranial pressure as evidenced by

a. spontaneous respirations within acceptable range (state specific highest and lowest rates for each child)
b. heart rate within acceptable range (state specific highest and lowest rates for each child)
c. pulse pressure within acceptable limits of 20 to 50 mm Hg
d. systolic pressure within acceptable range (state specific highest and lowest systolic pressures for each child)
e. lack of signs/symptoms of increased intracranial pressure (such as those listed under "Characteristics")

Possible Nursing Interventions

- Assess and record the following every 1 to 2 hours and PRN

  —neurologic vital signs (utilize Glasgow Coma Scale if available)
  —vital signs
  —signs/symptoms of increased intracranial pressure (such as those listed under "Characteristics"). Notify physician of any abnormalities.
  —central venous pressure (maintain between 4 and 8 mm Hg or within parameters ordered)

- Keep accurate record of intake and output. Restrict fluid intake as ordered.
- Elevate head of bed at a 30° angle (unless contraindicated); maintain head in a midline position.

- Keep environment as quiet as possible.
- Organize nursing care to minimize disturbance and stimulation of the child.
- Measure and record head circumference every shift.
- Ensure that anticonvulsants, osmotic agents, diuretics, steroids, muscle relaxants, antipyretics, and antibiotics are administered on schedule. Assess and record effectiveness and any side effects (such as electrolyte imbalance, GI bleeding, nausea, vomiting, and rash).
- Hyperventilate the child to decrease cerebral blood volume if indicated (i.e., sudden onset of symptoms of increased intracranial pressure).
- Maintain hypothermia if ordered for refractive increased intracranial pressure.

Evaluation for Charting

- State range of vital signs including CVP.
- Describe neurologic signs.
- Describe signs/symptoms of increased intracranial pressure (such as those listed under "Characteristics").
- Describe any therapeutic measures used to decrease intracranial pressure and their effectiveness.
- State intake and output.
- State whether medications were administered on schedule and describe any side effects.

Nursing Diagnosis IMPARIED GAS EXCHANGE

Definition Alteration in the exchange of oxygen and carbon dioxide in the lungs and/or at the cellular level

Possibly Related to	• Hyperventilation secondary to increased intracranial pressure
	• Respiratory arrest secondary to increased intracranial pressure
	• Use of paralyzing agents
	• Aspiration secondary to vomiting
Characteristics	Tachypnea
	Hypoxia
	Restlessness
	Confusion
	Inability to clear secretions
	Absence of spontaneous respirations/respiratory arrest
	Abnormal breath sounds including crackles, rhonchi, and wheezes

Expected Outcomes

Child will maintain adequate gas exchange as evidenced by

  a. clear and equal breath sounds bilaterally
  b. respiratory rate within acceptable range (state specific highest and lowest rates for each child)
  c. $PaCO_2$ between 20 and 25 mm Hg (alkalosis is thought to decrease cerebral blood volume)
  d. PaO_2 between 75 and 100 mm Hg
  e. absence of confusion and restlessness

Possible Nursing Interventions

• Assess and record the following every 1 to 2 hours and PRN

  —breath sounds
  —signs/symptoms of impaired gas exchange (such as those listed under "Characteristics")

• Assess and record arterial blood gas values as ordered. Notify physician of any abnormalities.

- Check ventilator setting (FiO2, Rate, PIP or TV, PEEP/CPAP) every 15 minutes. Record every 1 to 2 hours.
- Suction using sterile technique every 2 hours and PRN.
- Ensure that chest physiotherapy is being done effectively and on schedule.
- Ensure that antibiotics and muscle relaxants are administered on schedule. Assess and record effectiveness and any side effects (such as rash, diarrhea, tachycardia, or nausea/vomiting).
- Elevate head of bed at a 30° angle, unless contraindicated.

Evaluation for Charting

- Describe breath sounds.
- State highest and lowest respiratory rate.
- State whether there are any spontaneous respirations.
- State type of endotracheal tube used and ventilator settings.
- State frequency of suctioning and describe characteristics of secretions.
- Describe any signs/symptoms of impaired gas exchange (such as those listed under "Characteristics").
- State highest and lowest arterial blood gas values and state the ongoing physiological process (i.e., respiratory alkalosis).
- State whether chest physiotherapy was done on schedule. Describe child's response to chest physiotherapy and its effectiveness in improving gas exchange.
- State whether antibiotics and muscle relaxants were administered on schedule. Describe any side effects.

- State whether head of bed was elevated.

Nursing Diagnosis **POTENTIAL FOR INFECTION**

Definition Invasion of the body by pathogenic organisms

Possibly Related to
- Numerous invasive procedures
- Surgical procedure
- Wound contamination

Characteristics Fever
Redness
Swelling
Purulent drainage
Lethargy
Irritability
Foul odor
Change in level of consciousness
Opisthotonos
Positive Kernig and Brudzinski signs
Nuchal rigidity
Sluggish, dilated, or unequal pupils
Abnormal or decreased breath sounds
Cyanosis
Tachypnea
Tachycardia
Hypotension
Diaphoresis
Altered white blood cell count

Expected Outcomes Child will be free of infection as evidenced by

a. body temperature within acceptable range of 36.5 to 37.2° C
b. clean wound sites with minimal clear to serosanguinous drainage
c. age-appropriate reflexes
d. clear and equal breath sounds
e. respiratory rate within acceptable range (state specific highest and lowest rates for each child)

f. heart rate within acceptable range (state specific highest and lowest rates for each child)
g. blood pressure within acceptable range (state specific highest and lowest B/P for each child)
h. white blood cell count within normal limits (state specific highest and lowest counts for each child)
i. lack of signs/symptoms of infection such as those listed under "Characteristics"

Possible Nursing Interventions

- Assess and record every 1 to 2 hours and PRN

  —vital signs
  —neurologic signs
  —breath sounds
  —signs/symptoms of infection such as those listed under "Characteristics"

- Maintain good handwashing technique.
- Ensure that wound care is done using aseptic technique. Assess and record amount and characteristics of drainage.
- Obtain culture specimens (wound, blood, tracheal) if ordered. Check results and notify physician of any abnormalities.
- Check and record results of CBC. Notify physician if CBC results are out of the acceptable range.
- Ensure that chest physiotherapy is being done effectively and on schedule.
- Suction using sterile technique every 2 hours and PRN. Record amount and characteristics of secretions.

- Reposition child as indicated.
- Ensure that antibiotics and antipyretics are administered on schedule. Assess and record effectiveness and any side effects (such as diarrhea and rash).

Evaluation for Charting

- State range of vital signs.
- Describe neurologic signs and breath sounds.
- Describe wound site and amount and characteristics of any drainage.
- Describe any abnormal reflexes.
- State frequency of suctioning and describe amount and characteristics of secretions. Describe effectiveness of chest physiotherapy.
- State results of any cultures and/or CBC if available.
- Describe any signs/symptoms of infection (such as those listed under "Characteristics").
- State whether antibiotics and antipyretics were administered on schedule. Describe effectiveness and any side effects.
- State how often child was repositioned.

Related Nursing Diagnoses

FLUID AND ELECTROLYTE IMBALANCE related to cerebral edema secondary to neurosurgery

ALTERATION IN COMFORT: PAIN related to

a. wound sites
b. increased intracranial pressure
c. numerous invasive procedures

CHILD'S/FAMILY'S FEAR related to

a. frightening surgery
b. uncertain prognosis and sequelae

Medical Diagnosis

REYE SYNDROME

Pathophysiology

Reye syndrome, a multisystem disease, is characterized by acute encephalopathy and fatty infiltration of the viscera of the brain and liver; Reye syndrome almost always follows a viral illness (varicella, influenza A and B). Histological changes have also been seen in skeletal muscle, kidney, pancreas, and cardiac tissue. The specific cause of Reye syndrome is unknown. Current theory suggests that, at the cellular level, the mitochondria are targeted by this disease. The mitochondrial morphological and functional changes produced by Reye syndrome contribute not only to the failure of many organs but also to many biochemical abnormalities. For example, in the liver there is disruption of the cycle in which ammonia is converted to urea, resulting in hyperammonemia. Other biochemical abnormalities include elevated fatty and organic acids, elevated serum glutamic-oxaloacetic transaminase (SGOT) and serum glutamic-pyruvic transaminase (SGPT), and prolonged prothrombin time.

Reye syndrome occurs most often in children 6 to 12 years of age. Initial symptoms include malaise, nausea, vomiting, irritability, and personality/behavioral changes. The child's consciousness may then quickly deteriorate into varying degrees of coma.

Primary Nursing Diagnosis	**ALTERATION IN LEVEL OF CONSCIOUSNESS**
Definition	Reduced or impaired state of awareness; can range from mild to complete impairment
Possibly Related to	Increased intracranial pressure secondary to cerebral edema (vasogenic, hyperemic, or cytotoxic)
Characteristics	*Stage I* Drowsiness Lethargy Vomiting Normal serum ammonia level Brisk pupillary reaction Ability to follow commands Glasgow Coma Scale Score greater than 8 Increased liver enzyme activity *Stage II* Disorientation/agitation/delirium Combativeness Hyperventilation Tachycardia Stupor Purposeful response to pain Hyperactive reflexes Increased serum ammonia level Increased liver enzyme activity Glasgow Coma Scale Score of 6 to 8 *Stage III* Unresponsive Comatose Decorticate rigidity Hyperventilation Intact brainstem reflexes Dilated pupils/reactive to light Increased serum ammonia level Increased liver enzyme activity Glasgow Coma Scale Score of 5

Stage IV

Deepening coma

Decerebrate posturing

Loss of ocular reflexes

Large, fixed pupils

Doll's eyes

Minimal serologic evidence of liver dysfunction

Glasgow Coma Scale Score of 4

Stage V

Seizures

No withdrawal from painful stimuli

Absence of spontaneous respirations

Loss of deep tendon reflexes

Flaccidity

Liver function normal

Glasgow Coma Scale Score of 3 or below

Expected Outcomes

Child will maintain an appropriate level of consciousness as evidenced by

    a. pupils that are equal and react to light

    b. equal movement of all extremities

    c. age-appropriate reflexes

    d. age-appropriate response to pain

    e. alterness when awake

    f. oriented X3 (if age-appropriate)

    g. recognition of family members (if age-appropriate)

    h. age-appropriate developmental level (state individualized examples for each child)

    i. ability to perform age-appropriate activities of daily living (state individualized examples for each child)

Child will be free of signs/symptoms of increased intracranial pressure as evidenced by

a. spontaneous respirations within acceptable range (state specific highest and lowest rates for each child)
b. heart rate within acceptable range (state specific highest and lowest rates for each child)
c. pulse pressure within acceptable limits of 20 to 50 mm Hg
d. systolic pressure within acceptable range (state specific highest and lowest systolic pressure for each child)
e. lack of signs/symptoms of increased intracranial pressure (such as those listed under "Characteristics")

Possible Nursing Interventions

- Assess and record the following every 1 to 2 hours and PRN

  —neurologic vital signs (utilize Glasgow Coma Scale if available)
  —vital signs
  —signs/symptoms of increased intracranial pressure (such as those listed under "Characteristics"). Notify physician of any abnormalities.
  —central venous pressure (maintain between 4 and 8 mm Hg or within parameters ordered)

- Keep accurate record of intake and output. Restrict fluid intake as ordered (usually 2/3 to 3/4 maintenance).
- Elevate head of bed at a 30° angle; maintain head in midline position.
- Keep environment as quiet as possible.

- Organize nursing care to minimize disturbance and stimulation of the child.
- If intracranial catheter is in place,

  —monitor intracranial pressure every 15 minutes. Record every 1 to 2 hours and PRN.
  —notify physician if intracranial pressure is above 20 mm Hg (normal ICP, 5 to 12 mm Hg)
  —calculate and record cerebral perfusion pressure (mean arterial pressure minus intracranial pressure) every hour and PRN. Notify physician if perfusion pressure falls below 55 mm Hg.
  —monitor intracranial pressure while suctioning child. Hyperventilate child if intracranial pressure increases above 20 mm Hg; notify physician.

- Ensure that anticonvulsants, osmotic agents, diuretics, steriods, muscle relaxants, antipyretics, and antibiotics are administered on schedule. Assess and record their effectiveness and any side effects (such as electrolyte imbalance, GI bleeding, nausea, vomiting, and rash).
- Maintain hypothermia if ordered for refractive increased intracranial pressure.

Evaluation for Charting

- State range of vital signs including CVP.
- Describe neurologic signs.
- State highest and lowest intracranial and cerebral perfusion pressures.

- Describe signs/symptoms of increased intracranial pressure (such as those listed under "Characteristics").
- Describe any therapeutic measures used to decrease intracranial pressure and their effectiveness.
- State intake and output.
- State whether medications were administered on schedule. Describe any side effects.

Nursing Diagnosis   **IMPAIRED GAS EXCHANGE**

Definition   Alteration in the exchange of oxygen and carbon dioxide in the lungs and/or at the cellular level

Possibly Related to

- Hyperventilation secondary to increased intracranial pressure
- Respiratory arrest secondary to increased intracranial pressure
- Use of paralyzing agents
- Aspiration secondary to vomiting

Characteristics   Hyperventilation/respiratory alkalosis
Tachypnea
Hypoxia
Restlessness
Confusion
Inability to clear secretions
Absence of spontaneous respirations/respiratory arrest
Abnormal breath sounds including crackles, rhonchi, and wheezes

Expected Outcomes   Child will maintain adequate gas exchange as evidenced by

a. clear and equal breath sounds bilaterally
b. respiratory rate within acceptable range (state specific highest and lowest rates for each child)

**Possible Nursing
Interventions**

c. PaCO2 between 20 and 25 mm Hg (alkalosis is thought to decrease cerebral blood flow)
d. PaO2 between 75 and 100 mm Hg
e. absence of confusion and restlessness

- Assess and record the following every 1 to 2 hours and PRN

    —breath sounds
    —signs/symptoms of impaired gas exchange (such as those listed under "Characteristics")

- Assess and record arterial blood gas values as ordered. Notify physician of any abnormalities.
- Check ventilator settings (FiO2, Rate, PIP or TV, PEEP/CPAP) every 15 minutes. Record every 1 to 2 hours.
- Suction using sterile technique every 2 hours and PRN. Record amount and characteristics of secretions. Ensure that chest physiotherapy is being done effectively and on schedule.
- Ensure that antibiotics and muscle relaxants are administered on schedule. Assess and record effectiveness and any side effects (such as rash, diarrhea, tachycardia, or nausea/vomiting).
- Elevate head of bed at a 30° angle, unless contraindicated.

**Evaluation
for Charting**

- Describe breath sounds.
- State highest and lowest respiratory rates.
- State whether there are any spontaneous respirations.

- State type of endotracheal tube used and ventilator settings.
- State frequency of suctioning and describe characteristics of secretions.
- Describe any signs/symptoms of impaired gas exchange (such as those listed under "Characteristics").
- State highest and lowest arterial blood gas values and state the ongoing physiological process (i.e., respiratory alkalosis).
- State whether chest physiotherapy was done on schedule. Describe child's response to chest physiotheraphy and its effectiveness in improving gas exchange.
- State whether antibiotics and muscle relaxants were administered on schedule. Describe any side effects.
- State whether head of bed was elevated.

ALTERATION IN METABOLIC FUNCTION

Nursing Diagnosis

Definition Imbalance in the body of the utilization of specific biochemicals

Possibly Related to
- Disruption of the urea cycle
- Hepatic damage

Characteristics Hyperammonemia (vomiting, ataxia, tachypnea, coma)

Prolonged prothrombin time (bleeding from puncture sites or gums, blood in urine)

Increased SGOT

Increased SGPT

Increased lactate dehydrogenase (LDH)

Increased uric acid

Hypoglycemia

Hypocalcemia (tetany, hyperactive reflexes, convulsions)
Metabolic acidosis

Expected Outcomes

Child will have adequate metabolic function as evidenced by

a. ammonia within acceptable range of 15 to 45 μg/dl
b. prothrombin time within acceptable range of 12 to 14 seconds
c. SGOT within acceptable range of 10 to 40 IU/liter
d. SGPT within acceptable range of 5 to 35 IU/liter
e. LDH within acceptable range of 60 to 150 units
f. uric acid within acceptable range of 3 to 5 mg/dl
g. glucose within acceptable range of 60 to 120 mg/dl
h. calcium within acceptable range of 8.5 to 10.5 mg/dl
i. lack of metabolic acidosis
j. lack of signs/symptoms of metabolic dysfunction such as those listed under "Characteristics"

Possible Nursing Interventions

• Assess and record every 1 to 2 hours and PRN

—vital signs
—neurologic signs
—signs/symptoms of metabolic dysfunction such as those listed under "Characteristics"

• Assess and record laboratory values as indicated (usually every 4 to 6 hours). Notify physician of any abnormalities.

• Keep accurate record of intake and output.

- Assess and record IV fluids and condition of IV site every hour.
- Ensure that medications (Aqua-MEPHYTON, lactulose, neomycin, fresh frozen plasma, and calcium supplements) are administered on schedule if ordered. Assess and record their effectiveness and any side effects (such as diarrhea and arrhythmias).

Evaluation Charting

- State range of vital signs.
- State highest and lowest laboratory values.
- State intake and output.
- Describe condition of IV site.
- Describe any signs/symptoms of metabolic dysfunction (such as those listed under "Characteristics")
- Describe the effectiveness of any therapeutic measures used to correct metabolic dysfunction.

Related Nursing Diagnoses

FLUID VOLUME DEFICIT related to

a. vomiting
b. hyperventilation (insensible water loss)
c. diuretic therapy

ALTERATION IN NUTRITION: LESS THAN BODY REQUIREMENTS related to

a. vomiting
b. liver dysfunction

INEFFECTIVE FAMILY COPING related to

a. sudden serious illness of child, possibly fatal

b. multiple treatments and procedures
c. guilt from not having recognized
seriousness of symptoms earlier
d. uncertain prognosis and sequelae

Medical Diagnosis	# STATUS EPILEPTICUS
Pathophysiology	Status epilepticus is defined as a single seizure or series of seizures lasting 30 minutes or longer, during which consciousness does not return. Generalized tonic-clonic seizures are the most common, but the seizures may also be focal. At the cellular level, status epilepticus results when the membranes of the epileptiform cells in the brain do not restabilize.
Primary Nursing Diagnosis	## ALTERATION IN LEVEL OF CONSCIOUSNESS
Definition	Reduced or impaired state of awareness; can range from mild to complete impairment
Possibly Related to	• Cerebral hypoxia secondary to prolonged seizure activity • Cerebral edema secondary to prolonged seizure activity • Prolonged seizure activity secondary to —trauma —infection —metabolic disturbance —electrolyte disturbance —degenerative neurological disease —tumor —toxins —underlying cerebral malformations —withdrawal of anticonvulsants, alcohol, or other toxic agents, e.g., cocaine
Characteristics	Tonic-clonic (myoclonic) movements Cyanosis Grunting Apnea

Increased salivation
Eye rolling
Confusion
Staring into space
Incontinence of urine/stool
Change or loss of consciousness

Expected Outcomes

Child will be free of seizure activity.

Possible Nursing Interventions

- Assess for any early signs/symptoms (e.g., onset of uncontrollable activity) that may lead to seizure activity.
- Assess and record all seizure activity including

  —beginning and progression sequence
  —duration
  —type of movements
  —incontinence
  —level of consciousness

- If seizure activity does occur

  —stay with the child.
  —protect the child from injury.
  —keep side rails up and padded if child is in bed.
  —place child on flat, soft surface.
  —move sharp objects away from child.
  —loosen any restrictive clothing.
  —position child to prevent upper airway obstruction.
  —try to insert oral airway gently if child has not clamped down.
  —administer oxygen if ordered.
  —assist with intubation if necessary.

- Ensure that anticonvulsants, hypertonic glucose, calcium chloride, and calcium gluconate are administered as ordered.

Evaluation for Charting	• State range of vital signs.
	• Describe seizure activity.
	• Describe any therapeutic measures used to control the seizure activity and their effectiveness.
	• State whether medications were administered as ordered.

Nursing Diagnosis

IMPAIRED GAS EXCHANGE

Definition

Alteration in the exchange of oxygen and carbon dioxide in the lungs and/or at the cellular level

Possibly Related to

• Anoxia during seizure activity
• Aspiration secondary to seizure activity

Characteristics

Irregular, labored respirations
Grunting
Apnea
Choking
Cyanosis
Shallow respirations
Tachypnea
Dyspnea
Increased secretions

Expected Outcomes

Child will maintain adequate gas exchange as evidenced by

a. clear and equal breath sounds bilaterally
b. respiratory rate within acceptable range (state specific highest and lowest rates for each child)
c. lack of signs/symptoms of impaired gas exchange (such as those listed under "Characteristics")
d. arterial pH between 7.35 and 7.45
e. $PaCO_2$ between 35 and 45 mm Hg
f. PaO_2 between 75 and 100 mm Hg

**Possible Nursing
Interventions**

g. arterial bicarbonate level between 22 and 28 mEq/liter

- During seizure activity

    —roll patient into a side-lying position to maintain a patent airway and allow drainage of secretions.
    —try to insert an oral airway gently if child has not clamped down.
    —administer oxygen as ordered.
    —assist with intubation if necessary.
    —suction airway as indicated.

- If child is intubated

    —check ventilator settings (FiO2, Rate, PIP or TV, PEEP/CPAP) every 15 minutes. Record every 1 to 2 hours.
    —suction using sterile technique every 2 hours and PRN.

- Assess and record the following every 1 to 2 hours and PRN

    —breath sounds
    —color
    —signs/symptoms of impaired gas exchange (such as those listed under "Characteristics")
    —blood gas values. Report any abnormalities to the physician.

**Evaluation
for Charting**

- Describe any seizure activity and the effectiveness of any therapeutic measures used to control seizure activity.
- State type of endotracheal tube used and ventilator settings.
- State frequency of suctioning and characteristics of secretions.
- State highest and lowest arterial blood gas values and state the ongo-

ing physiologic process (i.e., respiratory acidosis).
- Describe any signs/symptoms of impaired gas exchange (such as those listed under "Characteristics") and the effectiveness of any measures used to improve gas exchange.
- Describe breath sounds and child's color.

Nursing Diagnosis **POTENTIAL FOR INJURY**

Definition Situation in which child sustains (or is at risk of sustaining) damage or harm

Possibly Related to Characteristics
Prolonged seizure activity
Alteration in level of consciousness
Pain
Hemorrhage
Swelling, edema
Open wounds

Expected Outcomes Child will be free of injury

Possible Nursing Interventions

- During seizure activity

  —do not attempt to restrain child or use force.
  —stay with child.
  —protect head from injury (place helmet on child if indicated).
  —loosen any restrictive clothing.
  —ease child onto a soft, flat surface

- Keep side rails up and padded, if child is in bed.
- Move sharp objects and furniture away from child.

Evaluation for Charting

- Describe any nursing interventions implemented and their effectiveness.
- Describe any signs/symptoms of injury noted after seizure activity (such

as those listed under "Characteristics").

Related Nursing Diagnoses

DECREASED CARDIAC OUPUT related to

a. seizure activity
b. anticonvulsant administration

CHILD'S FEAR related to

a. unpredicatable nature of seizure
b. embarrassment

DISTURBANCE IN SELF-CONCEPT related to

a. medication side effects
b. activity restrictions
c. interruption/failure in achieving developmental tasks

Medical Diagnosis	# CROUP, LARYNGOTRACHEOBRONCHITIS

Pathophysiology

"Croup" is a term used to describe a set of symptoms that result from swelling or obstruction in the area of the larynx. These symptoms include hoarseness, "barky" cough, and varying degrees of inspiratory stridor and respiratory distress. Laryngotracheobronchitis (LTB) is the most common of the croup syndromes that require hospitalization. LTB involves both the upper and the lower airways. Inflammation and edema begin in the glottic and subglottic areas and then progress down to the trachea and bronchi. Parainfluenza viruses, influenza viruses, and respiratory synticial viruses are the main viral agents that cause LTB. LTB most often affects children 3 months to 3 years of age.

Primary Nursing Diagnosis

INEFFECTIVE BREATHING PATTERN

Definition

A breathing pattern that results in oxygen insufficient to meet the cellular requirements of the body

Possibly Related to

A viral infection of the larynx, trachea, and bronchi

Characteristics

Inspiratory stridor
Hoarseness
"Barky" cough
Tachypnea
Dyspnea
Diminished breath sounds bilaterally
Crackles and rhonchi
Substernal and suprasternal retractions
Fever
Irritability and restlessness

Cyanosis (late sign)
Insidious onset

Expected Outcomes

Child will have an effective breathing pattern as evidenced by

a. clear and equal breath sounds bilaterally
b. respiratory rate within acceptable range (state specific highest and lowest rates for each child)
c. temperature of 36.5° to 37.2° C
d. lack of

—hoarseness
—inspiratory stridor at rest
—"barky" cough
—retractions
—extreme irritability and restlessness
—cyanosis

Possible Nursing Interventions

- Assess and record every 2 hours and PRN

—breath sounds with vital signs
—signs/symptoms of ineffective breathing pattern and increasing airway obstruction (such as those listed under "Characteristics")

- Administer cool mist by ordered route of delivery.
- Administer oxygen in the correct amount and route. Assess and record effectiveness of therapy. Be aware that over 40% oxygen may mask symptoms of increasing respiratory distress. Arterial blood gases may be indicated.
- Ensure that nebulized bronchodilators (such as racemic epinephrine) and antipyretics are administered on schedule. Steroids (such as dexa-

methasone) may be ordered, but their effectiveness remains controversial. Assess and record effectiveness and any side effects (such as tachycardia and GI disturbances).

- Deep suction only if it is specifically ordered. Suctioning may induce laryngospasms and cause further airway obstruction.

Evaluation for Charting

- Describe breath sounds.
- State highest and lowest respiratory rate and temperature.
- Describe any signs/symptoms of ineffective breathing pattern or increasing airway obstruction (such as those listed under "Characteristics").
- State whether cool mist was administered and the route of delivery. Describe effectiveness.
- State amount and route of oxygen delivery. Describe effectiveness.
- State whether medications were administered on schedule. Describe effectiveness and any side effects.
- State whether suctioning was needed. If so, describe any problems encountered during suctioning, the characteristics of the secretions, and the response of the child.

Nursing Diagnosis **FLUID VOLUME DEFICIT**

Definition A decrease in the amount of circulating fluid volume

Possibly Related to

- Respiratory difficulty
- Sore throat
- Increased insensible water loss from rapid respirations

Characteristics Anorexia

Inability to tolerate fluids by mouth

Vomiting
Tachypnea
Malaise
Dry mucous membranes
Poor skin turgor

Expected Outcomes

Child will have an adequate fluid volume as evidenced by

    a. adequate fluid intake, IV or oral (state exact amount of intake needed for each child)
    b. adequate urinary output (state specific highest and lowest outputs for each child)
    c. urine specific gravity between 1.008 and 1.020
    d. moist mucous membranes
    e. rapid skin recoil

Possible Nursing Interventions

- Keep accurate record of intake and output.
- Assess and record

    —IV fluids and condition of IV site every hour
    —signs/symptoms of fluid volume deficit (e.g., dry mucous membranes and poor skin turgor) every 2 hours and PRN

- Check and record urine specific gravity every void or as ordered.
- Give mouth care every 4 hours and PRN.

Evaluation for Charting

- State intake and output.
- Describe condition of IV site.
- Describe status of mucous membranes and skin turgor.
- State highest and lowest urine specific gravity.

Related Nursing Diagnoses

FEAR, CHILD'S related to

    a. respiratory distress
    b. unfamiliar surroundings
    c. forced contact with strangers
    d. treatments and procedures
    e. restraints

ACTIVITY INTOLERANCE related to

    a. respiratory difficulty
    b. fatigue
    c. confinement to mist area

ALTERATION IN NUTRITION: LESS THAN BODY REQUIREMENTS related to anorexia secondary to respiratory distress

INEFFECTIVE FAMILY COPING related to

    a. respiratory distress of child
    b. hospitalization of child

| Medical Diagnosis | **EPIGLOTTITIS** |

Pathophysiology

Epiglottitis is considered a medical emergency because of the possibility of complete airway obstruction from an enlarged epiglottis. Epiglottitis is characterized by inflammation and edema of the epiglottis, the aryepiglottic folds, and the false cords (supraglottic area). *Haemophilus influenzae* type glottitis, and it is isolated more frequently from the blood than from the larynx or trachea. Epiglottitis most often affects children aged 3 to 7.

Primary Nursing Diagnosis

IMPAIRED GAS EXCHANGE

Definition

Alteration in the exchange of oxygen and carbon dioxide in the lungs and/or at the cellular level

Possibly Related to

- An upper airway bacterial infection of the epiglottis
- Total airway obstruction secondary to edema of the epiglottis

Characteristics

Difficulty, swallowing or inability to swallow

Drooling of saliva

Muffled voice

Inspiratory stridor

Retractions

Decreased breath sounds bilaterally

Tachypnea

"Fish-mouth" breathing

Sitting upright, refusal to lie down, head craned forward, chin thrust out, tripod position

Fever

Hypoxia, hypercapnia, and acidosis

Cyanosis (late sign)

Anxious and frightened expression

Listlessness (late sign)

Red, sore, inflamed throat

Large, cherry-red, edematous epiglottis

Epiglottis as a large, rounded soft tissue
mass below the base of the tongue on
lateral neck x-ray

Abrupt onset

Absent cough

**Expected
Outcomes**

Child will have adequate gas exchange
as evidenced by

a. patent airway
b. clear and equal breath sounds
c. respiratory rate within acceptable
range (state specific highest and
lowest rate for each child)
d. ability to swallow
e. temperature of 36.5° to 37.2° C
f. lack of

—inspiratory stridor
—retractions
—cyanosis
—edema and discoloration of epiglottis
—extreme anxiety
—listlessness

g. appropriate-sized epiglottis on
neck x-ray
h. arterial pH of 7.35 to 7.45
i. PaCO2 between 35 and 45 mm
Hg
j. PaO2 between 75 and 100 mm Hg
k. arterial bicarbonate level between
22 to 28 mEq/L

**Possible Nursing
Interventions**

• Assess and record every 2 hours and
PRN

—breath sounds and vital signs

—signs/symptoms of impaired gas exchange or airway obstruction (such as those listed under "Characteristics")

- Before intubation

  —keep head of bed elevated at a 45° angle.
  —assess constantly for any signs/symptoms of increasing airway obstruction.
  —keep the following equipment at the bedside

    ☐ endotracheal and tracheostomy tubes
    ☐ oxygen equipment
    ☐ suction equipment

- After intubation (mechanical ventilation is ordinarily not necessary)

  —suction using sterile technique every 2 hours and PRN. Record amount and characteristics of secretions.
  —administer humidified air/oxygen in the amount ordered; record percentage of liter flow and route of delivery (usually via T-piece) every 2 hours; assess and record effectiveness of therapy.
  —if indicated, ensure that sedatives (such as chloral hydrate) are administered on schedule. Assess and record effectiveness.
  —restrain (elbow splints) according to hospital policy if indicated.

- Ensure that antibiotics (such as cephalosporins), steroids (such as hydrocortisone and dexamethasone), and antipyretics are administered on schedule. Assess and record effectiveness and any side effects (such as diarrhea, rash, and GI disturbances).

- Assess and record arterial blood gas values as ordered. Notify physician of any abnormalities.
- Encourage family members to stay if it helps to decrease the child's anxiety.

Evaluation for Charting

- Describe breath sounds.
- State highest and lowest respiratory rate and temperature.
- Describe any signs/symptoms of impaired gas exchange or airway obstruction (such as those listed under "Characteristics").
- State whether child was intubated. State type of endotracheal tube used. State how often child was suctioned and describe amount and characteristics of secretions.
- State amount and route of humidified air/oxygen delivered. Describe effectiveness.
- State highest and lowest arterial blood gas values and state the ongoing physiologic process (i.e., respiratory acidosis).
- State whether medications were administered on schedule. Describe effectiveness and any side effects.
- State whether family members stayed with the child and whether it helped to decrease the child's anxiety.

Nursing Diagnosis   **INEFFECTIVE THERMOREGULATION**

Definition   Instability of the child's body temperature

**Possibly
Related to**
- Bacterial invasion of the epiglottis
- Bacterial invasion of the bloodstream

Characteristics
Fever
Tachycardia
Hypotension
Tachypnea
Lethargy, irritability
Diaphoresis
Skin hot to touch
Flushed face
Increased white blood cell count
Decreased appetite

**Expected
Outcomes**
Child will be free of signs/symptoms of ineffective thermo-regulation as evidenced by

a. temperature of 36.5° to 37.2° C
b. heart rate, respiratory rate, and B/P with acceptable range (state highest and lowest parameters for each child)
c. skin dry and warm to touch
d. lack of lethargy and irritability
e. no decrease in appetite
f. white blood cell count within normal limits (state specific highest and lowest counts for each child)

**Possible Nursing
Interventions**
- Assess and record the following every 2 hours and PRN

  —temperature
  —vital signs
  —signs/symptoms of ineffective thermoregulation (such as those listed under "Characteristics")

- Give tepid sponge baths as indicated.
- Ensure that antibiotics (such as cephalosporins) and antipyretics are administered on schedule. Assess

and record effectiveness and any side effects (such as rash and diarrhea).

Evaluation for Charting

- State range of vital signs.
- Describe any signs/symptoms of ineffective thermoregulation (such as those listed under "Characteristics").
- Describe any successful therapeutic measures used to correct the child's hyperthermia.
- State whether medications were administered on schedule. Describe effectiveness and any side effects.

Related Nursing Diagnoses

FLUID VOLUME DEFICIT related to

  a. respiratory difficulty
  b. sore throat
  c. refusal to swallow
  d. insensible water loss from rapid respirations and increased temperature

FEAR, CHILD'S related to

  a. respiratory difficulty
  b. unfamiliar surroundings
  c. forced contact with strangers
  d. treatments and procedures

ALTERATION IN LEVEL OF CONSCIOUSNESS related to

  a. respiratory distress
  b. sedation

INEFFECTIVE FAMILY COPING related to

  a. hospitalization of child
  b. life-threatening nature of illness
  c. respiratory distress of child
  d. sudden onset of illness

Medical Diagnosis	# FOREIGN BODY ASPIRATION
Pathophysiology	A foreign body may be aspirated into any section of the airway, from the larynx to the bronchi. If a small object is aspirated, a wheeze is audible as the air passes around the obstructing object during both inspiration and expiration. A larger obstruction may result in obstructive emphysema, from inspired air being trapped distal to the obstruction. Air is neither inspired or expired when there is complete airway obstruction by an object and swollen mucosa. The air distal to the obstruction will soon absorb, resulting in an area of atelectasis. Because the right bronchus is straighter and shorter, it is the most common site of bronchial obstruction. Foreign body aspiration must be considered when an afebrile child has a sudden onset of respiratory distress.
Primary Nursing Diagnosis	## INEFFECTIVE AIRWAY CLEARANCE
Definition	Inability to clear secretions or objects from the airways
Possibly Related to	Airway obstruction by a small object (round candy, nut, coin, grape, meat, etc.)
Characteristics	Choking Rhonchi Wheezing Gagging Sudden, periodic coughing Periods during which child is asymptomatic for days or weeks after initial onset of symptoms ***Secondary Characteristics*** Fever

Dyspnea
Asymmetry of chest expansion
Decreased breath sounds over affected
   lung
Recurrent intractable pneumonia
Locational Characteristics
Larynx
Hoarseness
Croupy cough
Inspiratory stridor
Inability to vocalize
Trachea
Cough
Hoarseness
Dyspnea
Cyanosis
Bronchus
Cough
Blood-tinged sputum
Dyspnea

Expected Outcomes

Child will be able to clear airways adequately as evidenced by

   a. clear and equal breath sounds bilaterally
   b. symmetry of chest expansion
   c. thin, clear secretions
   d. absence of

      —choking
      —coughing
      —wheezing
      —gagging
      —rhonchi
      —inspiratory stridor
      —dyspnea
      —hoarseness
      —cyanosis

   e. ability to vocalize
   f. temperature within acceptable range of 36.5° to 37.2° C

Possible Nursing Interventions

- Assess and record the following every 2 hours and PRN

    —breath sounds and vital signs
    —signs/symptoms of ineffective airway clearance (such as those listed under "Characteristics)

- Assess and record amount and characteristics of any pulmonary secretions.
- Ensure that chest physiotherapy is being done effectively and on schedule.
- Check and record results of chest x-ray when indicated.
- Ensure that antibiotics and/or bronchodilators are administered on schedule. Assess and record effectiveness and any side effects (such as rash, diarrhea, tachycardia, or nausea/vomiting).
- Prepare child for surgical treatments such as bronchoscopy.
- Explain to the child's family any indicated procedure and its rationale.

Evaluation for Charting

- Describe breath sounds.
- Describe any sign/symptoms of ineffective airway clearance.
- State whether the chest physiotherapy treatments were effective in moving the foreign object out of the airways.
- State highest and lowest temperatures.
- State results of chest x-ray if appropriate.
- State whether antibiotics and/or bronchodilators were administered

on schedule. Describe any side effects.
- Describe child's level of tolerance for any surgical procedure that might have been done, such as bronchoscopy.
- If procedure was done, state whether infant showed any signs of improvement after the procedure.

Nursing Diagnosis

Definition

FLUID VOLUME DEFICIT

A decrease in the circulating fluid volume

Possibly Related to

- Dyspnea
- Choking

Characteristics

Decreased ability to tolerate PO fluids due to dyspnea

Dry mucous membranes

Poor skin tugor

Expected Outcomes

Child will have an adequate fluid volume as evidenced by

    a. adequate fluid intake, IV or oral (state exact amount of intake needed for each child)

    b. adequate urinary output (state specific highest and lowest outputs for each child)

    c. urine specific gravity of 1.008 to 1.020

    d. moist mucous membranes

    e. rapid skin recoil

Possible Nursing Interventions

- Keep accurate record of intake and output.
- Assess and record

    —IV fluids and condition of IV site every hour

    —signs/symptoms of fluid volume deficit (e.g., dry mucous membranes and poor skin tugor) every 2 hours and PRN

- Check and record urine specific gravity every void or as ordered.
- Give mouth care every 4 hours and PRN.

Evaluating for Charting

- State intake and output.
- Describe condition of IV site.
- Describe status of mucous membranes and skin turgor.
- State highest and lowest urine specific gravity.

Nursing Diagnosis **FEAR, CHILD'S**

Definition Feeling of apprehension resulting from a known cause

Possibly Related to

- Respiratory distress
- Unfamiliar surroundings
- Forced contact with strangers
- Treatments and procedures
- Hospitalization

Characteristics
Restlessness
Constant crying
Tachypnea
Tachycardia
Diaphoresis

Expected Outcomes
Child will exhibit only a minimal amount of fear as evidenced by

a. appropriate relating to family members
b. ability to rest and sleep between treatments and procedures
c. lack of constant crying
d. respiratory rate within acceptable range (state specific highest and lowest rates for each child)

e. heart rate within acceptable range (state specific highest and lowest rates for each child)
f. lack of diaphoresis

Possible Nursing Interventions

- Decrease child's fear when possible by

  —encouraging family members to stay with child
  —encouraging family members to participate in the care of the child
  —trying to have the same staff members care for the child
  —talking to child and explaining procedures and treatments along with why they are necessary
  —trying to spend extra time with the child when family members are unable to be present
  —encouraging family members to bring in familiar articles and toys from home

- Initiate age-appropriate play therapy if indicated.
- Assess and record any physiologic signs/symptoms of fear (e.g., increased respiratory rate, increased heart rate, and/or diaphoresis) when taking vital signs.

Evaluation for Charting

- State whether child manifested fear and describe any successful measures used to help alleviate the fear.
- State whether the child's fear decreases if family members stay and participate in the child's care.
- State highest and lowest respiratory and heart rates.
- State whether diaphoresis was present.

Nursing Diagnosis	**GUILT, PARENTAL/FAMILY**
Definition	A state or condition in which the individual accepts blame, either appropriate or inappropriate
Possibly Related to	• Accidental nature of child's illness • Discomfort child is experiencing • Delay in seeking health care
Characteristics	Verbalization of blame Overprotectiveness of ill child Anger Irritability

Expected Outcomes	Parents/family will be able to deal with guilt feelings appropriately, as evidenced by
	
	  a. expressing fears/concerns to members of the health care team
	  b. participating in child's care when possible
	  c. accepting help when indicated

Possible Nursing Interventions	• Encourage family to ventilate and express feelings of guilt; give positive reinforcement for doing so. • Praise any positive family/child interaction observed. • Encourage family to participate in child's care when possible. • Encourage and assist family in seeking outside help/counseling when appropriate.
Evaluation for Charting	• Describe any concerns/fears expressed by family. • State whether family paricipated in child's care. • Describe any successful measures used to help decrease family's guilt feelings.

Related Nursing Diagnoses

• State whether family sought outside counseling.

POTENTIAL FOR INFECTION related to

a. aspiration
b. invasive procedures

KNOWLEDGE DEFICIT, PATENTAL/ FAMILY related to care and safety of a young child

Medical
Diagnosis

NEAR-DROWNING

Pathophysiology

The second most common cause of accidental death in children is drowning, with teenage boys and toddlers being at highest risk. Ten to 15% of drownings are "dry," denoting laryngospasm without evidence of aspiration. Eighty-five to 90% of drownings are associated with aspiration and are considered "wet." The complications of drowning are directly related to the volume and composition of the water that is aspirated and the degree of hypoxia. Fresh water drownings are more common than salt water drownings. In fresh water drowning, hypoxia results from intrapulmonary right-to-left shunting caused by surfactant alteration and atelectasis and, if a massive amount of water is aspirated, water intoxication may occur, resulting in hyponatremia, hemodilution with hemolysis, hyperkalemia, and hypervolemia. In salt water drowning, hypoxia results from intrapulmonary right-to-left shunting caused by surfactant washout and/or plasma leak into the alveoli and hypovolemia may occur secondary to plasma loss into the alveoli if massive amounts of fluid are aspirated.

Primary Nursing
Diagnosis

IMPAIRED GAS EXCHANGE

Definition

Alteration in the exchange of oxygen and carbon dioxide in the lungs and/or at the cellular level

Possibly
Related to

- Hypoxemia
- Transient hypercapnia
- Laryngospasm

- Breath holding
- Aspiration
- Intrapulmonary shunt
- Atelectasis
- Pulmonary edema
- Altered properties of pulmonary surfactant

Characteristics   Apnea
Diminished breath sounds
Cyanosis
Retractions
Nasal flaring
Stridor
Wheezing
Cough
Crackles
Rhonchi
Respiratory acidosis
Increased pulmonary secretions
Lung infections
Pneumothorax
Tachypnea
Tachycardia
Bradycardia

Expected Outcomes

Child will maintain adequate gas exchange as evidenced by

a. clear and equal breath sounds bilaterally
b. symmetrical chest expansion
c. respiratory rate within acceptable range (state specific highest and lowest rates for each child)
d. lack of

—cyanosis
—nasal flaring
—stridor
—retractions
—cough

e. arterial pH between 7.35 and 7.45

f. PaCO2 between 35 and 45 mm Hg
g. PaO2 between 75 and 100 mm Hg
h. arterial bicarbonate level between 22 and 28 mEq/liter
i. clear chest x-ray
j. heart rate within acceptable range (state specific highest and lowest rates for each child)
k. body temperature maintained between 36.5° and 37.2° C

Possible Nursing Interventions

- Assess and record the following every 1 to 2 hours and PRN

  —breath sounds
  —color
  —signs/symptoms of impaired gas exchange (such as those listed under "Characteristics")

- Assess and record arterial blood gas values as ordered. Notify physician of any abnormalities.
- Check ventilator settings (FiO2), Rate, PIP or TV, PEEP/CPAP) every 15 minutes. Record every 1 to 2 hours.
- Suction using sterile technique every 2 hours and PRN.
- Ensure that chest physiotherapy is being done effectively and on schedule.
- Ensure that antibiotics and/or bronchodilators are administered on schedule. Assess and record effectiveness and any side effects (such as rash, diarrhea, tachycardia, or nausea/vomiting).
- Elevate head of bed at a 30° angle, unless contraindicated.

Evaluation for Charting

- Describe breath sounds.
- Describe child's color.
- State range of vital signs.
- State whether there are any spontaneous respirations.
- State type of endotracheal tube used and ventilator settings.
- State frequency of suctioning and describe characteristics of secretions.
- Describe any signs/symptoms of impaired gas exchange (such as those listed under "Characteristics").
- State highest and lowest arterial blood gas values and state the ongoing physiologic process (i.e., respiratory acidosis).
- State whether chest physiotherapy was done on schedule. Describe child's response to chest physiotherapy and its effectiveness in improving gas exchange.
- State whether antibiotics and/or bronchodilators were administered on schedule. Describe any side effects.
- State whether head of bed was elevated.

ALTERATION IN LEVEL OF CONSCIOUSNESS

Nursing Diagnosis

Definition
Reduced or impaired state of awareness; can range from mild to complete impairment

Possibly Related to

- Increased intracranial pressure secondary to cerebral edema resulting from hypoxia and/or ischemia
- Cerebral perivascular hemorrhage

Characteristics
Lethargy
Stupor

Restlessness
Irritability
Pupillary changes
Apnea
Seizures
Headache
Decreased response to pain
Decreased response to verbal commands
Hypothermia
Hyperthermia
Abnormal posturing
Altered Babinski reflex
Doll's eyes
Vomiting
Bradycardia
Widening pulse pressure
Elevated systolic pressure
Respiratory arrest
Cardiac arrest

Expected Outcomes

Child will maintain an appropriate level of consciousness as evidenced by

    a. pupils that are equal and react to light
    b. equal movement of all extremities
    c. normal-pitched cry
    d. age-appropriate reflexes
    e. age-appropriate response to pain
    f. alertness when awake
    g. orientation ×3 (if age-appropriate)
    h. recognition of family members (if age-appropriate)
    i. age-appropriate developmental level (state individualized examples for each child)
    j. ability to perform age-appropriate activities of daily living (state individualized examples for each child)

Child will be free of signs/symptoms of increased intracranial pressure as evidenced by

   a. spontaneous respirations within acceptable range (state specific highest and lowest rates for each child)
   b. heart rate within acceptable range (state specific highest and lowest rates for each child)
   c. pulse pressure within acceptable limits of 20 to 50 mm Hg
   d. systolic pressure within acceptable range (state specific highest and lowest systolic pressures for each child)
   e. temperature within acceptable range of 35.6° to 37.2° C
   f. lack of signs/symptoms of increased intracranial pressure (such as those listed under "Characteristics")

Possible Nursing Interventions

- Assess and record the following every 1 to 2 hours and PRN

   —neurologic vital signs (utilize Glasgow Coma Scale if available)
   —vital signs
   —signs/symptoms of increased intracranial pressure (such as those listed under "Characteristics"). Notify physician of any abnormalities.

- Keep accurate record of intake and output. Restrict fluid intake as ordered (usually 1/2 to 2/3 maintenance).
- Elevate head of bed at a 30° angle; mintain head in midline position.

- Maintain child's body temperature between 35.6° and 37.2° C.
- Keep environment as quiet as possible.
- Organize nursing care to minimize disturbance and stimulation of the child.
- If intracranial catheter is in place,

    —monitor intracranial pressure every 15 minuts. Record every 1 to 2 hours and PRN.
    —notify physician if intracranial pressure is above 20 mm Hg.
    —calculate and record cerebral perfusion pressure (mean arterial pressure minus intracranial pressure) every hour and PRN.
    —monitor intracranial pressure while suctioning child. Hyperventilate child if intracranial pressure increases above 20 mm Hg; notify physician.

- Ensure that anticonvulsants, osmotic agents, diuretics, steroids, muscle relaxants, antipyretics, and antibiotics are administered on schedule. Assess and record effectiveness and any side effects (such as electrolyte imbalance, GI bleeding, nausea, vomiting, and rash).

Evaluation for Charting

- State range of vital signs and describe neurologic signs.
- State highest and lowest intracranial pressures and cerebral perfusion pressures.
- Describe signs/symptoms of increased intracranial pressure (such as those listed under "Characteristics").

- Describe any therapeutic measures used to decrease intracranial pressure and their effectiveness.
- State intake and output.
- State whether medications were administered on schedule. Describe any side effects.

Nursing Diagnosis	## ALTERATION IN FLUID AND ELECTROLYTE BALANCE
Definition	Disturbance in the amount of body fluid and disturbance in the values of body electrolytes
Possibly Related to	• Central nervous system injury resulting in an increase or decrease in the production of antidiuretic hormone • Respiratory acidosis • Metabolic acidosis • Decreased renal perfusion • Aspiration of fresh water • Aspiration of salt water

Characteristics	*Fresh Water* (Hypotonic Solution)
	Hypervolemia
	Hemodilution
	Hyperkalemia
	    Weakness
	    Paralysis
	    Oliguria
	    EKG changes: spiked T waves, flattened P wave, ventricular dysrhythmias
	Hyponatremia
	    Weakness
	    Delirium
	    Seizures
	    Oliguria with water retention
	    Specific gravity will vary, less than 1.010 with diuresis and greater than 1.010 with water retention

***Salt Water* (Hypertonic Solution)**

Hypovolemia

Hemoconcentration

Hypokalemia

   Muscle irritability or weakness

   Paresthesias

   Hypotension

   Rapid, weak, irregular pulse

   EKG changes: flat T waves, peaked P
     wave

Hypernatremia

   Flushed skin

   Agitated, restless state

   Dry mucous membranes

   Oliguria

   Specific gravity will vary, less than
     1.010 if diabetes insipidus is pre-
     sent, greater than 1.015 if water
     loss is nonrenal

Other

Metabolic acidosis

Tachycardia

Edema

Weak peripheral pulse

Sunken eyes

Cool extremities

Prolonged capillary refill, longer than 2
   to 3 seconds

Poor skin turgor

**Expected
Outcomes**

Child will resume fluid and electrolyte
balance as evidenced by

    a. adequate urine output (state spe-
       cific highest and lowest outputs
       for each child, 1 to 2 ml/kg/hour)

    b. receipt of the ordered amount of
       fluid intake (state exact amount al-
       lowed for each child)

    c. urine specific gravity between
       1.008 to 1.020

    d. lack of edema

e. age-appropriate blood pressure (state specific highest and lowest pressures for each child)

f. normal sinus rhythm

g. heart rate within acceptable range (state highest and lowest rates for each child)

h. serum potassium of 3.5 to 5.0 mEq/liter

i. serum sodium of 138 to 145 mEq/liter

j. serum chloride of 101 to 108 mEq/liter

k. serum carbon dioxide of 18 to 27 mEq/liter

l. absence of signs/symptoms of hyponatremia, hypernatremia, hypokalemia, and hyperkalemia (such as those listed under "Characteristics")

m. rapid skin recoil

n. strong and equal peripheral pulses

o. skin warm to touch

p. brisk capillary refill, within 2 to 3 seconds

Possible Nursing Interventions

- Assess and record the following every 1 to 2 hours and PRN

  —vital signs

  —signs/symptoms of fluid or electrolyte imbalance (such as those listed under "Characteristics"). Report abnormalities to the physcian.

  —laboratory values as indicated. Report abnormalities to the physician.

  —IV fluids and condition of IV site every hour. Perform IV site care as directed by institutional policy.

- Evaluate and record results of EKG strips.
- Keep accurate record of intake and output.
- Check and record specific gravity every void or as ordered.
- Dipstick urine for blood, sugar, and protein; record.
- Monitor and record weight as ordered.
- Foley care as per institutional policy.
- Give mouth care every 4 hours and PRN.

Evaluating for Charting

- State intake and output.
- Describe characteristics of urine.
- State range of dipstick and specific gravity results.
- State range of vital signs including blood pressure.
- State current laboratory values. If any were abnormal, state action taken and effectiveness or results of action taken..
- Describe any signs/symptoms of fluid or electrolyte imbalance.
- State weight and determine whether it has increased or decreased from previous weight.

INEFFECTIVE THERMOREGULATION: HYPOTHERMIA

Nursing Diagnosis

Definition Instability of child's body temperature; core body temperature of less than 35° C

Possibly Related to

- Prolonged cold water immersion
- Central nervous system injury

Characteristics Temperature of less than 35° C
Bradycardia

Dysrhythmias, especially ventricular fibrillation

Skin cool to touch

Sluggish capillary refill, longer than 2 to 3 seconds

Bradypnea/apnea

Areflexia

Unresponsiveness

Dilated pupils

Muscle rigidity

Expected Outcomes

Child will be free of signs/symptoms of hypothermia as evidenced by

a. temperature of 35.6° to 37.2° C
b. respiratory rate within acceptable range (state specific highest and lowest rates for each child)
c. heart rate within acceptable range (state specific highest and lowest rates for each child)
d. brisk capillary refill, within 2 to 3 seconds
e. skin warm to touch
f. rapid skin recoil
g. alterness and orientation when awake
h. age-appropriate reflexes

Possible Nursing Interventions

- Assess and record the following every 1 to 2 hours and PRN

  —temperature
  —vital signs
  —signs/symptoms of hypothermia (such as those listed under "Characteristics").

- For children with a core temperature of less than 29° C, provide the following if ordered

  —heated, humidified oxygen
  —warmed IV fluids

—warmed gastric and/or peritoneal lavage fluids (may be warmed to 40° C)

- For children with a core temperature of 29° C to 32° C, provide the following if ordered

  —warmed IV fluids
  —heated, humidified oxygen
  —heating blankets

- For children with a core temperature greater than 32° C, rewarm with heating blankets as ordered.
- When rewarming child, increase body core temperature by 1° C per hour.
- Keep child away from air drafts.
- Keep child dry; change as soon as possible after elimination.

Evaluation for Charting

- State range of vital signs.
- State temperature of heating blanket.
- Describe any signs/symptoms of hypothermia (such as those listed under "Characteristics").
- Describe any successful therapeutic measures used to correct the child's hypothermia.

Related Nursing Diagnoses

GUILT, PARENTAL/FAMILY related to

a. knowledge deficit
b. accidental nature of child's illness
c. discomfort child is experiencing
d. lack of child supervision

POTENTIAL FOR INFECTION related to

a. aspiration
b. invasive procedures

STATUS ASTHMATICUS

Pathophysiology

Asthma, also called reactive airway disease, is a recurrent, reversible respiratory process. It is characterized by increased responsiveness of the trachea, bronchi, and bronchioles to various stimuli producing bronchospasm, mucosal edema, and hypersecretion of mucus. Hyperinflation of the lungs also occurs, resulting in air trapping.

Status asthmaticus develops when an acute asthma attack progresses to the point where it does not respond to vigorous therapeutic measures including two to three inhaled or parenteral treatments of sympathomimetics. There is little air exchange, and carbon dioxide is retained. Pulmonary vasoconstriction with intrapulmonary shunting occurs because the child is hypoxic and in respiratory and metabolic acidosis. In extreme cases the child may develop cor pulmonale (right ventricular hypertrophy secondary to pulmonary hypertension) or pulmonary edema.

Primary Nursing Diagnosis

IMPAIRED GAS EXCHANGE

Definition

Alteration in the exchange of oxygen and carbon dioxide in the lungs and/or at the cellular level

Possibly Related to

- Spasms of the smooth muscle of the bronchi and bronchioles
- Accumulation of tenacious secretions
- Edema of the mucous membranes of the airways

<table>
<tr><td></td><td>• Allergies</td></tr>
<tr><td></td><td>• Viral infections</td></tr>
<tr><td>Characteristics</td><td>Wheezing (inspiratory and/or expiratory)</td></tr>
</table>

Characteristics Wheezing (inspiratory and/or expiratory)

Decreased air entry on auscultation (silent chest)

Tachypnea

Retractions

Use of accessory muscles

Nasal flaring

Dyspnea

Prolonged expiratory time

Cough

Cyanosis

Hyperinflation of lungs on chest x-ray

Crackles, rhonchi

Hypoxia

Hypercarbia

Acidosis

Anxiety

Fatigue

Change in level of consciousness, restlessness, irritability, and lethargy

Expected Outcomes Child will have adequate gas exchange as evidenced by

   a. clear and equal breath sounds bilaterally

   b. respiratory rate within acceptable range (state specific higest and lowest rate for each child)

   c. lack of

     —retractions

     —use of accessory muscles

     —nasal flaring

     —cough

     —cyanosis

     —extreme anxiety

     —extreme fatigue

d. clear chest x-ray with appropriate AP diameter
e. arterial pH of 7.35 to 7.45
f. PaCO2 between 35 and 45 mm Hg
g. PaO2 between 75 and 100 mm Hg
h. arterial bicarbonate level of 22 to 28 mEq/liter
i. level of consciousness appropriate for age

Possible Nursing Interventions

- Assess and record every 1 to 2 hours and PRN

  —breath sounds
  —respiratory rate
  —signs/symptoms of impaired gas exchange (such as those listed under "Characteristics")

- Assess and record arterial blood gas values when indicated and report any abnormalities to the physician.
- Assess and record serum theophylline levels when indicated and report any abnormalities to the physician.
- Assess and record results of chest x-ray when indicated.
- Administer oxygen in the correct amount and route. Assess and record effectiveness of therapy.
- Ensure that chest physiotherapy is being done on schedule. Record effectiveness of treatment.
- Keep head of bed elevated at a 30° to 45° angle.
- Ensure that bronchodilators (such as theophylline, epinephrine, isoproterenol, and terbutaline) and steroids (hydrocortisone, prednisone) are administered on schedule. Assess and record effectiveness and any side ef-

fects (such as tachycardia and GI disturbances).

Evaluation for charting
- Describe breath sounds.
- State highest and lowest respiratory rate.
- Describe any signs/symptoms of impaired gas exchange (such as those listed under "Characteristics").
- State highest and lowest arterial blood gas values and state the ongoing physiologic process (i.e., respiratory acidosis).
- State the serum theophylline level and any therapeutic changes made.
- State amount and route of oxygen delivery. Describe effectiveness.
- Describe effectiveness of chest physioatherapy treatments.
- State whether the head of the bed was kept elevated.
- State whether medications were administered on schedule. Describe effectiveness and any side effects.

Nursing Diagnosis | **DECREASED CARDIAC OUTPUT**

Definition | A decrease in the amount of blood that leaves the left ventricle

Possibly Related to
- Hypoxia
- Acidosis
- Side effects of drug therapy

Characteristics | Tachycardia
Dysrhythmias
Cyanosis
Weak peripheral pulses
Pulsus paradoxus

Expected Outcomes | Child will maintain an adequate cardiac output as evidenced by

a. heart rate within acceptable range (state specific highest and lowest rates for each child)
b. normal sinus rhythm
c. lack of cyanosis
d. strong and equal peripheral pulses
e. lack of pulsus paradoxus

Possible Nursing Interventions

- Assess and record every 2 hours and PRN
  —heart rate
  —peripheral pulses
  —blood pressure
  —any signs/symptoms of decreased cardiac output (such as those listed under "Characteristics").
- Evaluate and record results of EKG strips at least once/shift.
- Keep accurate record of intake and output.

Evaluation for Charting

- State highest and lowest apical rate and B/P.
- Describe quality of peripheral pulses.
- Describe any signs/symptoms of decreased cardiac output (such as those listed under "Characteristics").
- Document EKG interpretation.
- State intake and output.

Nursing Diagnosis **FEAR, CHILD'S**
Definition Feeling of apprehension resulting from a known cause

Possibly Related to

- Respirato;ry distress
- Treatments and procedures
- Unfamiliar surroundings
- Forced contact with strangers
- Hospitalization

Characteristics	Restlessness
	Tachypnea
	Tachycardia
	Diaphoresis
	Uncooperativeness

Expected Outcomes

Child will exhibit only a minimal amount of fear as evidenced by

    a. appropriate relating to family members

    b. ability to rest and sleep betwen treatments and procedures

    c. respiratory rate within acceptable range (state specific highest and lowest rates for each child)

    d. heart rate within acceptable range (state specific highest and lowest rates for each child

    e. lack of diaphoresis

    f. cooperation with treatments and procedures

Possible Nursing Interventions

• Decrease child's fear when possible by

    —encouraging family members to stay with child

    —encouraging family members to participate in the care of the child

    —trying to have the same staff members care for the child

    —talking to child and explaining procedures and treatments along with why they are necessary

    —trying to spend extra time with the child when family members are unable to be present

    —encouraging family members to bring in familiar articles and toys from home

- Initiate age-appropriate play therapy if indicated.
- Assess and record any physiologic signs/symptoms of fear (e.g., tachypnea, tachycardia, and/or diaphoresis) when taking vital signs.
- Ensure that call light is available (if appropriate).
- Organize nursing care to minimize disturbance of the child.

Evaluation for Charting

- State whether child manifested fear and describe any successful measures used to help alleviate the fear.
- State whether the child's fear decreases if family members stay and participate in the child's care.
- State highest and lowest respiratory and heart rates.
- State whether the child was diaphoretic.
- State whether the child was cooperative during treatments and procedures.
- State whether the child was able to rest and sleep between treatments and procedures.

Related Nursing Diagnoses

FLUID VOLUME DEFICIT related to

a. respiratory distress
b. increased insensible water loss from rapid respiratory rate

ACTIVITY INTOLERANCE related to dyspnea

INEFFECTIVE FAMILY COPING related to

a. repeated hospitalization of child
b. respiratory distress of child

CARDIOVASCULAR SURGERY, POSTOPERATIVE CARE

Pathophysiology

Cardiovascular surgery is most often performed on children for the palliation or correction of congenital heart defects. Closed heart surgery involves structures associated with the heart and does not require that the child be placed on cardiopulmonary bypass. Examples of closed heart surgery include patent ductus ligation, pulmonary artery banding, and repair of coarctation of the aorta. In open heart surgery, an incision is made into the myocardium to reach the internal cardiac structures that need repair and, therefore, cardiopulmonary bypass is required. Examples of open heart surgery include septal defect repairs, repair of the tetralogy of Fallot, and correction of transposition of the great vessels.

During the postoperative period, continual and thorough assessments are required for prompt recognition and treatment of problems. There are numerous potential postoperative complications of cardiovascular surgery, which can involve any bodily system.

Primary Nursing Diagnosis

DECREASED CARDIAC OUPTUT

Definition

A decrease in the amount of blood that leaves the left ventricle

Possibly Related to

Surgical complicaitons such as

- thrombus
- ineffective circulation
- interference with electrical conduction

	• cardiac muscle dysfunction
	• hemorrhage
	• cardiac tamponade
	• dysrhythmias
	• tachycardia or bradycardia
	• decreased oxygenation
	• hypovolemia
	• hypervolemia
Characteristics	Tachycardia/bradycardia

Dysrhythmias

Hypotension/hypertension

Unequal, decreased, or absent peripheral pulses

Prolonged capillary refill, longer than 2 or 3 seconds

Murmur, gallop, rub, click

Cool, pale skin

Increased chest tube drainage (more than 3ml/kg/hour)

Decreased cardiac index (less than 2.5 liters/min/m² or a downhill trend)

Decreased urinary output (less than 0.5 to l ml/kg/hour)

Decreased hematocrit and hemoglobin

Hypovolemia/hypervolemia

Prolonged PT and PTT

Right atrial pressures (or CVP) less than 4 mm Hg or more than 12 to 15 mm Hg

Expected Outcomes

Child will maintain an adequate cardiac output as evidenced by

a. heart rate within acceptable range (state specific highest and lowest rates for each child)

b. blood pressure within acceptable range (state specific highest and lowest blood pressures for each child)

c. normal sinus rhythm

d. strong and equal peripheral pulses

e. brisk capillary refill, within 2 to 3 seconds
f. skin warm to touch
g. lack of murmur, gallop, rub, click
h. chest tube drainage of less than 3 ml/kg/hour
i. PTT within acceptable range of 11 to 16 seconds (normal values will be set by each laboratory)
j. PTT within acceptable range of 30 to 45 seconds
k. cardiac index within acceptable range of 2.5 to 4 liters/min/m^2
l. right atrial pressure (or CVP) within acceptable range of 4 to 8 mm Hg
m. Hct and Hgb within acceptable ranges (state specific highest and lowest values for each child)
n. adequate urine output (state specific highest and lowest output for each child; normal, one to 2 ml/kg/hour)

Possible Nursing Interventions

- Assess and record every 1 to 2 hours and PRN

  —apical rate and blood pressure
  —any signs/symptoms of decreased cardiac output (such as those listed under "Characteristics")
  —right atrial pressure of (or CVP), left atrial pressure, pulmonary artery pressure, and pulmonary capillary wedge pressure readings
  —peripheral pulses
  —capillary refill
  —amount and characteristics of chest tube drainage. Notify physician of excessive drainage.

- Evaluate and recod results of EKG strips at least once/shift.
- Compare vital signs with electronic monitoring devices at least once/shift.
- Keep accurate record of intake and output.
- Assess and record condition of dressing and/or incision site every shift and PRN. Notify physician of excessive drainage.
- Transfuse blood products to maintain adequate CVP and Hct/Hgb. Assess, record, and report any signs/symptoms of transfusion reaction (such as chills, fever, difficulty breathing).
- Ensure that cardiac drugs (digoxin, dopamine) are administered on schedule if ordered. Assess and record effectivenes and any side effects (such as bradycardia and decreased urine output).
- Use sterile technique when changing any of the invasive monitoring lines.
- Maintain identification and integrity of pacer wires if present. If pacemaker is in use, not pacer spikes on EKG strip and record rate, sensitivity, and milliamps.
- Ensure that chest tube system is intact and that negative pressure is maintained. Strip chest tubes to maintain patency as ordered. Record site of chest tube(s).

Evaluation for Charting

- State highest and lowest apical rate and B/P.
- Describe any signs/symptoms of decreased cardiac output (such as those listed under "Characteristics").

- State highest and lowest values for each of the following
  a. right atrial pressure (or CVP)
  b. left atrial pressure
  c. pulmonary artery pressure
  d. pulmonary capillary wedge pressure
  e. cardiac output/index
- Document EKG interpretation.
- State intake and output.
- Describe any therapeutic measures used to increase cardiac output, their effectiveness, and child's response.
- Describe condition of dressing and incision site.
- State highest and lowest hourly chest tube drainage.
- Describe amount and characteristics of chest tube drainage. State location of chest tube(s) and amount and type of suction.

Nursing Diagnosis   **IMPAIRED GAS EXCHANGE**
Definition   Alteration in the exchange of oxygen and carbon dioxide in the lungs and/or at the cellular level

Possibly Related to
- Decreased cardiac output
- Loss of surfactant during cardiopulmonary bypass
- Surgical invasion of the chest
- Surgical complications such as
  —atelectasis
  —pneumothorax
  —hemothorax
  —pleural effusion
  —pneumonia

Characteristics   Tachypnea
Dyspnea
Retractions
Cyanosis

Crackles
Restlessness
Agitation
Decreased breath sounds
Respiratory acidosis/hypercapnia
Hypoxemia
Respiratiory alkalosis/hypocapnia
Atelectasis
Nasal flaring
Unequal chest excursion
Hypoventilation
Decreased chest expansion

Expected Outcomes

Child will have adequate gas exchange as evidenced by

a. respiratory rate within acceptable range (state specific highest and lowest rates for each child)
b. clear and equal breath sounds biliaterally
c. clear chest x-ray
d. lack of

—retractions
—restlessness/agitation
—cyanosis
—nasal flaring

e. adequate chest expansion
f. symmetrical chest excursion
g. arterial pH of 7.35 to 7.45
h. PaCO2 of 35 to 45 mm Hg
i. PaO2 of 75 to 100 mm Hg
j. arterial bicarbonate level of 22 to 28 mEq/liter

Possible Nursing Interventions

• Assess and record every 2 hours and PRN

—breath sounds with respiratory rate

—signs/symptoms of impaired gas exchange (such as those listed under "Characteristics")

- Administer oxygen in the correct amount and route. Assess and record effectiveness of therapy.
- Elevate head of bed at a 30° angle.
- Assess and record arterial blood gas values as ordered. Notify physician of any abnormalities.
- Check ventilator settings (FiO2, Rate, PIP or TV, PEEP/CPAP) every 15 minutes. Record every 1 to 2 hours.
- Suction using sterile technique every 2 hours and PRN. Record amount and characteristics of secretions.
- Ensure that chest physiotherapy is being done effectively and on schedule. Record effectivness of treatment.
- Ensure that antibiotics and analgesiscs (morhpine) are administered on schedule. Assess and record effectiveness and any side effects (such as rash, diarrhea, and respiratory depression).
- Assess and record results of chest x-ray when indicated.
- Assist child with coughing and deep breathing, i.e., use of bedside spirometer, when indicated.

Evaluation for Charting

- Describe breath sounds.
- State highest and lowest respiratory rates.
- Describe any signs/symptoms of impaired gas exchange (such as those listed under ("Characteristics").
- State amount and route of oxygen delivery. Describe effectiveness.
- State whether head of bed was elevated.

- State highest and lowest arterial blood gas values and state the ongoing physiological process (i.e., respiratory acidosis).
- State type of endotracheal tube used and ventilator settings.
- State frequency of suctioning and describe amount and characteristics of secretions.
- State whether chest physiotherapy was done on schedule. Describe child's response to chest physiotherapy and its effectiveness in improving gas exchange.
- State whether antibiotics and analgesics were administered on schedule. Describe effectiveness and side effects noted.

Related Nursing Diagnoses

ALTERATION IN COMFORT related to

    a. surgical procedure
    b. fear
    c. procedures/treatment

POTENTIAL FOR INFECTION related to

    a. surgical procedure
    b. intubation
    c. invasive monitoring

FLUID VOLUME EXCESS related to surgical complications

INEFFECTIVE FAMILY COPING related to

    a. child's surgery
    b. child's hospitalization
    c. fear of child dying
    d. lack of support system
    e. expense of procedure

CONGESTIVE HEART FAILURE

Pathophysiology

Congestive heart failure (CHF) is not a disease in itself. CHF refers to a set of clinical signs and symptoms that indicate that the heart is unable to pump blood adequately to meet the body's metabolic demands. Heart failure may be right-sided or left-sided, but most often progresses to involve both sides.

In right-sided failure, because of dysfunction of the right ventricle, the right ventricular end-diastolic pressure rises resulting in increased central venous pressure and increased systemic venous engorgement, which may then lead to systemic congestion and edema.

Pulmonary venous engorgement and increased pressure in the left atrium occur when the left ventricular end-diastolic pressure rises because of left ventricular failure. The increased pulmonary pressure causes fluid to leak form the pulmonary capillaries into the interstitial spaces, resulting in pulmonary edema.

Congenital heart defects are the most common cause of CHF in children. CHF occurs most frequently during the child's first year of life. The goals in the treatment of CHF are to decrease the cardiac workload and to promote adequate cardiac output.

Primary Nursing Diagnosis

DECREASED CARDIAC OUTPUT

Definition

A decrease in the amount of blood that leaves the left ventricle

Possibly Related to	• Fluid volume overload
	• Pulmonary hypertension
	• Increased flow of blood to the lungs
	• Congenital heart defect
	• Acquired heart defect
	• Myocarditis
	• Myopathies
	• Noncardiovascular diseases (such as respiratory disease, anemia, metabolic disorders, and endocrine disorders)
Characteristics	Tachycardia
	Dyspnea
	Tachypnea
	Crackles
	Mottled skin
	Cyanosis
	Pale, cool skin
	Hepatosplenomegaly
	Cardiomegaly on chest x-ray
	Edema (peripheral, periorbital, sacral, and scrotal)
	Diaphoresis (especially over head and neck)
	Hypotension
	Rapid, weak peripheral pulses
	Prolonged capillary refill, longer than 2 to 3 seconds
	Narrow pulse pressure
	Weakness
	Extreme irritability
	Feeding difficulty
	Fatigue
	Gallop rhythm
	Decreased urinary output (less than 0.5 to 1 ml/kg/hour)
	Growth rate slower than normal
	Distended neck veins in older children

Expected Outcomes

Child will maintain an adequate cardiac output as evidenced by

  a. heart rate within acceptable range (state specific highest and lowest rates for each child)
  b. blood pressure within acceptable range (state specific highest and lowest blood pressures for each child)
  c. pulse pressure within acceptable limits of 20 to 50 mm Hg
  d. normal sinus rhythm
  e. strong and equal peripheral pulses
  f. brisk capillary refill, within 2 to 3 seconds
  g. skin warm to touch
  h. clear and equal breath sound bilaterally
  i. appropriate heart size on chest x-ray
  j. adequate urine output (state specific highest and lowest outputs for each child, 1 to 2 ml/kg/hour)
  k. steady progress on growth curve
  l. lack of signs/symptoms of decreased cardiac output (such as those listed under ("Characteristics")

Possible Nursing Interventions

• Assess and record every 2 hours and PRN

  —apical rate, blood pressure, and respiratory rate
  —any signs/symptoms of decreased cardiac output (such as those listed under ("Characteristics")

• Evaluate and record results of EKG strips.

- Keep accurate record of intake and output.
- Ensure that cardiac drugs (digoxin) are administered on schedule. Assess and record effectiveness and signs/symptoms of toxicity (such as bradycardia and vomiting). Assess and record apical rate for one full minute before giving digoxin. Do not give medication if apical rate is below 100 beats/minute or as orders indicate.
- Monitor and record digoxin levels. Notify physician if levels are out of the stated range.
- Ensure that diuretics (furosemide, spironolactone) are administered on schedule. Assess and record effectiveness and any side effects (such as hypokalemia and dehydration).
- Elevate head of bed to 30°.
- Organize nursing care to allow child uninterrupted rest periods.

Evaluation for Charting
- State highest and lowesxt apical rates, respiratory rates, and B/P.
- Describe cardiac rhythm and breath sounds.
- Describe any signs/symptoms of decreased cardiac output (such as those listed under ("Characteristics").
- Document EKG interpretation.
- State intake and output.
- State whether cardiac drugs and diuretics were given on schedule. Describe effectiveness and any side effects.
- State digoxin levels. If levels were out of the stated range, describe any measures required.
- State whether head of bed was elevated.

- State whether child had uninterrupted rest periods.

Nursing Diagnosis	**INEFFECTIVE BREATHING PATTERN**
Definition	A breathing pattern that results in oxygen insufficient to meet the cellular requirements of the body
Possibly Related to	• Decreased cardiac output • Pulmonary hypertension • Increased flow of blood to the lungs. • Congenital heart defect
Characteristics	Tachypnea Dyspnea Retractions Fatigue Pallor/mottling Cyanosis Crackles Expiratory grunt Nasal flaring Using of accessory muscles Infant head bobbing Dry hacking cough Shortness of breath Orthopnea Activity intolerance
Expected Outcomes	Child will have an effective breathing pattern as evidenced by

a. respiratory rate within acceptable range (state specific highest and lowest rates for each child)
b. clear and equal breath sounds bilaterally
c. lack of

—retractions/nasal flaring/expiratory grunt

—cough

—use of accesory muscles

—fatigue/activity intolerance
—cyanosis/pallor/mottling

Possible Nursing Interventions

- Assess and record every 2 hours and PRN

  —breath sounds with vital signs
  —signs/symptoms of ineffective breathing pattern (such as those listed under("Characeristics")

- Administer oxygen in the correct amount and route. Assess and record effectiveness of therapy.
- Elevate head of bed to 30°.
- Ensure that chest physiotherapy is being done effectively and on schedule. Record effectiveness and child's response to treatment.
- Suction using sterile technique as indicated. Record amount and characteristics of secretions.

Evaluation for Charting

- Describe breath sounds.
- State highest and lowest respiratory rate.
- Describe any signs/symptoms of ineffective breathing pattern (such as those listed under "Characteristics")
- State amount and route of oxygen delivery. Describe effectiveness.
- State whether head of bed was elevated.
- State whether chest physiotherapy was done on schedule. Describe effectiveness of chest physiotherapy and child's response.
- State frequency of suctioning and describe amount and characteristics of secretions.

Nursing Diagnosis	**FLUID VOLUME EXCESS**
Definition	Increased intravascular fluid volume, which can lead to interstitial fluid overload
Possibly Related to	Edema secondary to decreased cardiac output
Characteristics	Edema (periorbital, peripheral, sacral, scrotal)
	Decreased urinary output, less than 0.5 to 1 ml/kg/hour
	Weight gain
	Hypertension/hypotension
	Increased urine specific gravity (greater than 1.020)
	Crackles
	Hepatosplenomegaly
	Ascites

Expected Outcomes

Child will resume fluid balance as evidenced by

a. lack of edema or ascites
b. adequate urine output (state specific highest and lowest outputs for each child; 1 to 2 ml/kg/hour
c. blood pressure within acceptable range (state highest and lowest pressures for each child)
d. lack of rapid weight gain
e. urine specific graivity of 1.008 to 1.020
f. clear and equal abreath sounds bilaterally
g. lack of hepatosplenomegaly

Possible Nursing Interventions

- Keep an accurate record of intake and output. Ensure that child does not exceed maximal intake ordered. Record characteristics of urinary output.

- Check and record urine specific gravity every void or as ordered.
- Assess and record every 2 hours and PRN

  —blood pressure
  —breath sounds
  —signs/symptoms of fluid volume excess

- Assess and record amount and location of edema once/shift
- Weigh child on same scale (usually every 8 to 12 hours).
- Ensure that diuretics (furosemide, spironolactone) are administered on schedule. Before the administration of any ordered diuretic, check the most recent serum electrolyte values. If hypokalemia is present, notify physician before administering diuretic. Assess and record effectiveness and any side effects (such as hypokalemia and dehydration).

Exvaluation for Charting

- State intake and output.
- State highest and lowest urine specific gravity.
- State highest and lowest blood pressure.
- Describe breath sounds.
- Describe any signs/symptoms of fluid volume excess.
- Describe amount and location of edema.
- State child's weight and determine whether it has increased or decreased from the previous weight.
- State whether diuretics were administered on schedule. State most recent serum potassium level. Describe effectiveness and any side effects.

Related Nursing Diagnoses

ALTERATION IN NUTRITION: LESS THAN BODY REQUIREMENT related to

a. respiratory distress
b. decreased energy level
c. feeding difficulty

ACTIVITY INTOLERANCE related to

a. decreased cardiac output
b. respiratory distress
c. decreased energy

INEFFECTIVE FAMILY COPING related to

a. hospitalization of child in critical care unit
b. illness involving major body organ
c. added stress of chonic illness on family system

PAROXYSMAL ATRIAL TACHYCARDIA

Pathophysiology

Paroxysmal atrial tachycardia (PAT) is one of the most common dysrhythmias in children, occurring most frequently in 1- to 3-month old infants. PAT is a rapid, regular heart beat (above 200 beats/minute in infants) arising from an atrial or nodal (supraventricular) focus. The QRS complex is usually narrow. PAT may end spontaneously or with an increase in vagal tone. Measures used to icnrease vagal tone include the Valsalva maneuver, gagging, massaging the carotid sinus, or activating the diving reflex by submerging the child's face in ice water. Therapeutic drugs include verapamil, propranolol, and digitalis. When vagal stimulation or durg therapy fails to break the attack, cardioversion may be used. A child who has prolonged episodes of PAT may develop congestive heart failure within 24 to 48 hours.

Primary Nursing Diagnosis

DECREASED CARDIAC OUTPUT

Definition

A decrease in the amount of blood that leaves the left ventricle

Possibly Related to

Supraventricular tachycardia secondary to

- underlying heart disease, congenital or acquired
- myocarditis
- systemic infection
- drug toxicity
- status/postintraatrial cardiovascular surgery or cardiac catheterization

- electrolyte or metabolic imbalance
- stress
- cardiac tumors
- chest trauma
- unknown cause

Characteristics Tachycardia (160 to 200 beats/minute in children and adolescents, 200 to 300 beats/minute in infants)

Dyspnea

Palpitations

Hypostension

Rapid weak peripheral pulses

Prolonged capillary refill, longer than 2 to 3 seconds

Narrow QRS complex

Weakness

Extreme irritablility

Feeding difficulty

Pale, cool skin

Expected Outcome Child will maintain an adequate cardiac output as evidenced by

a. heart rate within acceptable range (state specific highest and lowest rates for each child)
b. blood pressure within acceptable range (state specific highest and lowest blood pressures for each child)
c. normal sinus rhythm
d. strong and equal peripheral pulses
e. brisk capillary refill, within 2 to 3 seconds
f. skin warm to touch
g. lack of

   —dyspnea
   —palpitations
   —weakness
   —extreme irritability

—feeding difficulty
—paleness

Possible Nursing Interventions

• Assess and record every 2 hours and PRN

  —apical rate and blood pressure
  —any signs/symptoms of decreased cardiac output (such as those listed under "Characteristics")

• Evaluate and record results of EKG strips
• Locate and have available cardioversion equipment.
• Keep accurate record of intake and output.
• Ensure that IV line is patent (for emergency medication administration).
• Ensure that antiarrhythmics (verapamil, propranolol) are administered on schedule if ordered. Assess and record effectiveness and any side effects (such as bradycardia and transient hypotension).
• Assist with any needed procedures/treatments (such as vagal stimulation or cardioversion). Assess and record effectiveness and child's response to any procedures/treatments.

Evaluation for Charting

• State highest and lowest apical rate and B/P.
• Describe any signs/symptoms of decreased cardic output (such as those listed under "Characteristics")
• Document EKG interpretaion.
• State intake and output.
• Describe any therapeutic measures used to increase cardiac output, their effectiveness, and child's response.

Nursing Diagnosis	**INEFFECTIVE BREATHING PATTERN**
Definition	A breathing pattern that results in oxygen insufficient to meet the cellular requirements of the body

Possibly Related to Characteristics

Decreased cardiac output
Tachypnea
Dyspnea
Retractions
Fatigue
Pallor
Cyanosis
Crackles
Venous congestion on chest x-ray

Expected Outcomes

Child will have an effective breathing pattern as evidenced by

a. respiratory rate within acceptable range (state specific highest and lowest rates for each child)
b. clear and equal breath sounds bilaterally
c. clear chest x-ray
d. lack of

—retractions
—fatigue
—cyanosis
—pallor

Possible Nursing Interventions

- Assess and record every 2 hours and PRN

—breath sounds with vital signs
—signs/symptoms of ineffective breathing pattern (such as those listed under "Charateristics")

- Administer oxygen in the correct amount and route. Assess and record effectivness of therapy.
- Elevate head of bed at a 30° angle.

**Evaluation
for Charting**

- Describe breath sounds.
- State highest and lowest respiratory rates.
- Describe any signs/symptoms of ineffective breathing pattern (such as those listed under "Characteristics").
- State amount and route of oxygen delivery. Describe effectiveness.
- State whether head of bed was elevated.

**Related Nursing
Diagnoses**

ALTERATION IN NUTRITION: LESS THAN BODY REQUIREMENTS related to

a. increased metabolic rate
b. feeding difficulty

FEAR, CHILD'S/PARENTAL related to

a. sudden onset of symptoms
b. treatments/procedures

KNOWLEDGE DEFICIT relate to

a. unknown cause of arrhythmia
b. unfamiliar treatments/procedures

ACTIVITY INTOLERANCE related to decreased cardiac output

Medical Diagnosis	# ABDOMINAL SURGERY, POSTOPERATIVE CARE
Pathophysiology	Abdominal surgery may be required for the correction, care, or repair of gastrointestinal anomalies, traumatic lesions, or malignancies. Common pediatric gastrointenstinal problems requiring abdominal surgery include pyloric stenosis, duodenal malformation, malrotation/midgut volvulus, intussusception, acute appendicitis, and trauma.
	Postoperatively, most pediatric patients who have had abdominal surgery are able to return to a general pediatric unit. If there are significant perioperative complications, such as shock, hemorrhage, sepsis, electrolyte imbalance, or respiratory problems, the child may need intensive care for stabilization and close observation.
Primary Nursing Diagnosis	## FLUID VOLUME DEFICIT (INTRAVASCULAR)
Definition	A decrease in the volume of circulating fluid
Possibly Related to	• Dehydration secondary to vomiting/diarrhea • Hemorrhage • Third spacing of body fluid
Characteristics	Tachycardia Hypotension Hypovolemia/decreased CVP Abdominal distention Prolonged absence of bowel sounds Diarrhea/vomiting Dry mucous membranes Poor skin turgor Sunken fontanel

Decreased urinary output
Increased specific gravity

Expected Outcomes

Child will have an adequate fluid volume as evidenced by

    a. adequate IV fluid intake (state exact amount of intake needed for each child)
    b. adequate urinary output (state specific highest and lowest outputs for each child; normal, 1 to 2 ml/kg/hours.
    c. heart rate and blood pressure within acceptable range (state specific highest and lowest parameters for each child)
    d. CVP of 4 to 8 mm Hg
    e. nondistended abdomen
    f. bowel sounds
    g. lackof diarrhea/vomiting
    h. moist mucous membranes
    i. rapid skin recoil
    j. flat fontanel
    k. urine specific gravity of 1.008 to 1.020

Possible Nursing Interventions

- Keep accurate record of intake and output.
- Keep NPO.
- Assess and record

    —IV fluids and condition of IV site every hour
    —signs/symptoms of fluid volume deficit (such as those listed under "Characteristics") every 2 hours and PRN
    —heart rate, B/P, and CVP every 2 hours and PRN
    —bowel sounds every 2 hours and PRN

- Measure and record abdominal girth every shift.
- Ensure that nasogastric tube is patent and connected to low intermittent suction. Irrigate as ordered.
- If third spacing of fluid is present, ensure that colloids followed by diuretics are administered as ordered. Assess and record effectiveness.
- Check and record urine specific gravity every void or as ordered.

Evaluation for Charting

- State intake and output.
- Describe condition of IV site.
- State highest and lowest heart rate and B/P.
- Describe any signs/symptoms of fluid volume deficit (such as those listed under "Characteristics").
- Describe bowel sounds.
- State current abdominal girth and determine whether it has increased or decreased since the previous measurement.
- Describe amount and characteristics of nasogastric drainage.
- Describe any therapeutic measures used to maintain adequate fluid volume and their effectiveness.
- State highest and lowest urine specific gravity values.

Nursing Diagnosis

POTENTIAL FOR INFECTION

Definition

Invasion of the body by pathogenic organisms

Possibly Related to

- Surgical procedure and incision
- Numerous invasive procedures
- Wound contamination

Characteristics

Fever or hypothermia
Abdominal pain/tenderness

Abdominal distention/rigidity
Lethargy/malaise
Foul odor
Redness
Swelling
Purulent drainage
Increased gastric drainage
Watery stools
Vomiting
Altered white blood cell count
Tachycardia/bradycardia
Hypotension
Tachypnea
Abnormal or decreased breath sounds
Diaphoresis

**Expected
Outcomes**   Child will be free of infection as evidenced by

a. body temperature within acceptable range of 36.5° to 37.2° C
b. lack of abdominal pain/tenderness
c. nondistended abdomen
d. clean wound sites with minimal clear to serosanguinous drainage
e. white blood cell count within normal limits (state specific highest and lowest counts for each child)
f. heart rate within acceptable range (state specific highest and lowest B/P for each child)
g. blood pressure within acceptable range (state specific highest and lowest B/P for each child)
h. respiratory rate within acceptable range (state specific highest and lowest rates for each child)
i. clear and equal breath sounds
j. lack of signs/symptoms of infections (such as those listed under "Characteristics")

**Possible Nursing
Interventions**
Assess and record every 1 to 2 hours
and PRN

    —vital signs
    —breath sounds
    —signs/symptoms of infection such
      as those listed under "Characteris-
      tics"

- Maintain good handwashing technique.
- Ensure that wound care is done using
  aseptic technique. Assess and record
  amount and characteristics of drainage.
- Obtain culture specimens (wound,
  blood) if ordered. Check results and
  notify physician of any abnormalities.
- Check and record results of CBC.
  Notify physician if CBC results are
  out of the acceptable range.
- Ensure that chest physiotherapy is
  being done effectively and on schedule, if ordered.
- Suction using sterile technique every
  2 hours and RPN. Record amount
  and characteristics of secretions.
- Reposition child as indicated.
- Ensure that antibiotics and antipyretics are administered on schedule. Assess and record effectiveness and any
  side effects (such as diarrhea and
  rash).

**Evaluation
for Charting**
- State range of vital signs.
- Describe breath sounds.
- Describe wound sites and amount
  and characteristics of any drainage.
- State results of any cultures and/or
  CBC if available.

- Describe any signs/symptoms of infection (such as those listed under "Characteristics").
- Describe effectiveness of chest physiotherapy.
- State frequency of suctioning and describe amount and characteristics of secretions.
- State how often child was repositioned.
- State whether antibiotics and antipyretics administered on schedule? Describe effectiveness and any side effects noted?

Related Nursing Diagnoses

ELECTROLYTE IMBALANCE related to fluid volume deficit

ALTERATION IN COMFORT related to

a. surgical incision
b. numerous invasive procedure

INEFFECTIVE BREATHING PATTERN related to

a. fluid volume deficit
b. abdominal distention
c. potential for infection

INEFFECTIVE FAMILY COPING related to

a. surgical procedure
b. child's hospitalization
c. emergency nature of illness

Medical Diagnosis

ACUTE GLOMERULONEPHRITIS

Pathophysiology

The specific pathophysiology of glomerulonephritis remains uncertain. Current theory suggests that the glomerulonephritis results from injuries to the glomerulus. One type of injury is caused by antigen-antibody complexes that affix themselves in Bowman's capsule of the kidney, resulting in a proliferative and exudative process (immune complex disease). Injury can also occur when antibodies are directed against antigens on the glomerular basement membrane (antiglomerular basement membrane disease).

The antigen-antibody complexes cause obstruction, inflammation, and edema in the kidney. The glomerular endothelial and epithelial cells proliferate and the affected area of the kidney is infiltrated by white blood cells. Renal capillary permeability increases and there is renal vascular spasm. These processes lead to decreased glomerular filtration. Water and sodium are retained, causing increased intravascular and interstitial fluid volume. A child with glomerulonephritis experiences hematuria, proteinuria, oliguria, edema, and hypertension.

Poststreptococcal glomerulonephritis is the most common type of glomerulonephritis. Viruses, pharmacological or toxic agents, and autoimmune diseases (i.e., lupus) may also be underlying causes of glomerulonephritis.

Primary Nursing Diagnosis	**FLUID VOLUME EXCESS**
Definition	An increase in the amount of circulation fluid volume
Possibly Related to	• Poststreptococcal infection • Antigen-antibody reaction • Pathological changes in the glomeruli
Characteristics	Oliguria Hematuria (coke-colored urine) Proteinuria Edema (especially periorbital) Hypertension Headache Abdominal pain Fever Lethargy Sudden weight gain Increased BUN Hepatomegaly
Expected Outcomes	Child will resume fluid balance as evidenced by

    a. adequate urine output (state specific highest and lowest outputs for each child; normal, 1 to 2 ml/kg/hour

    b. clear, pale yellow urine

    c. blood pressure within acceptable range (state specific highest and lowest blood pressures for each child)

    d. temperature of 36.5° to 37.2° C

    e. BUN between 5 and 18 mg/dl

    f. lack of

      —proteinuria
      —edema
      —headache
      —abdominal pain
      —lethargy

—sudden weight gain
—hepatomegaly

Possible Nursing Interventions

- Keep accurate record of intake and output. Be sure that child does not exceed maximal intake ordered. Document characteristics of urinary output.
- Assess and record

  —signs/symptoms of fluid volume excess (such as those listed under "Characteristics") every 2 hours and PRN
  —amount and location of edema at least once/shift
  —temperature and blood pressure every 2 hours and PRN
  —laboratory values as indicated. Report abnormalities to the physician.

- Weigh child daily on the same scale at the same time of day.
- Ensure that diuretics (such as furosemide) and antihypertensive medications (such as hydralazine) are administered on schedule. Assess and record effectiveness and any side effects (such as headache, nausea/vomiting, diarrhea, and tachycardia).

Evaluation for Charting

- State intake and output.
- Describe characteristics of urine output.
- Describe any signs/symptoms of fluid volume excess (such as those listed under "Characteristics").
- Describe amount and location of edema.
- State highest and lowest temperature and B/P.

- State child's weight and determine whether it has increased or decreased since the previous weighing.
- State whether medications were administered on schedule. Describe effectiveness and any side effects.

ALTERATION IN LEVEL OF CONSCIOUSNESS

Nursing Diagnosis

Definition

Reduced or impaired state of awareness; can range from mild to complete impairment

Possibly Related to

- Complication of hypertensive encephalopathy
- Electrolyte imbalance

Characteristics

Headache
Nausea/vomiting
Irritability
Lethargy
Seizures
Coma

Expected Outcomes

Child will maintain an appropriate level of consciousness as evidenced by

a. alertness when awake
b. orientation ×3 (if age-appropriate)
c. recognition of family members (if age-appropriate)
d. lack of

—headache
—nausea/vomiting
—irritability
—lethargy
—seizure activity

Possible Nursing Interventions

- Assess and record

—neurologic vital signs every 4 hours and PRN

—signs/symptoms of alteration in level of consciousness (such as those listed under "Characteristics") every 4 hours and PRN

- Organize nursing care to minimize disturbance and stimulation of the child.
- Assess and record all seizure activity including

  —beginning and progression sequence
  —duration
  —type of movements
  —incontinence
  —level of consciousness

- If seizure activity does occur

  —stay with the child.
  —protect the child from injury.
  —keep side rails up and padded if child is in bed.
  —place child on flat soft surface.
  —move sharp objects away from the child.
  —loosen any restrictive clothing.
  —position child to prevent upper airway obstruction.
  —try to insert oral airway gently if child has not clamped down.
  —administer oxygen if ordered.
  —assist with intubation if necessary.

Evaluation for Charting

- Describe neurologic vital signs.
- Describe any signs/symptoms of alteration in level of consciousness (such as those listed under "Characteristics").
- Describe any seizure activity.
- If seizures did occur, describe any therapeutic measures used to control

the seizure activity and their effectiveness.

Nursing Diagnosis

DISTURBANCE IN SELF-CONCEPT: BODY IMAGE

Definition A condition in which the child has a negative view of self

Possibly Related to
- Edema
- Sudden weight gain

Characteristics Verbalization about displeasure in body
Refusal to look into mirror
Refusal to participate in care
Decreased interest in appearance

Expected Outcomes Child will indicate acceptance of body image as evidenced by

a. verbalization of a positive body image
b. ability to look in mirror
c. willingness to participate in care
d. developmentally appropriate interest in appearance (state specific activities for each child)

Possible Nursing Interventions
- Assess and record child's and/or family's ability to accept altered body image.
- Encourage child and/or family to participate in care when possible.
- Encourage child to maintain usual state of grooming and appearance.

Evaluation for Charting
- Describe the child's and/or family's ability to accept altered body image.
- Describe any methods successful in helping child and/or family cope with child's altered body image.
- State whether child and/or family was willing to participate in care.

Related Nursing Diagnoses

- State whether child showed appropriate interest in his/her appearance.

DECREASED CARDIAC OUTPUT related to

a. hypertension
b. fluid volume excess

ALTERATION IN NUTRITION: LESS THAN BODY REQUIREMENTS related to sodium and protein restriction

ALTERATION IN PATTERNS OF URINARY ELIMINATION related to altered glomerular function

ACUTE RENAL FAILURE

The term acute renal failure (ARF) denotes a clinical situation in which renal function is impaired. During ARF the body's biochemical balance is disturbed, resulting in altered fluid volume regulation, the accumulation of nitrogenous waste products, electrolyte imbalance, and acid-base imbalance. In some renal diseases, dehydration may occur as the kidney loses its ability to concentrate the urine and large amounts of water are eliminated. In most renal diseases, as the disease process progresses and the glomerular filtration rate decreases, renin and aldosterone are stimulated, and sodium and water are retained, resulting in decreased urine output and edema.

Azotemia, an elevation in the blood urea nitrogen (BUN) and creatinine levels, occurs as renal function decreases and nitrogenous wastes are retained. Several electrolyte imbalances exist, including hyponatremia, hyperkalemia, hypocalcemia, and hyperphosphatemia. Metabolic acidosis occurs secondary to the retention of fixed acid.

ARF can be a direct result of kidney disease or it can be a complication of numerous systemic disorders. The causes of ARF are classified into prerenal, renal, and postrenal depending on the location of the primary disorder.

Prerenal causes of ARF usually create a hypoperfusion of the kidneys. There is a decrease in the glomerular filtration rate, but rarely is the renal parenchyma damaged. Therefore, renal function can usually be restored once the primary disorder is treated. Dehydration is a common cause of prerenal ARF.

Renal causes of ARF, such as chronic prerenal or postrenal problems, damage part of the nephron (glomeruli, tubules, or vessels). Damage may also be secondary to glomerular diseases (such as glomerulonephritis), ischemia (such as acute tubular necrosis), or nephrotoxins, and there is always some resultant renal insufficiency.

Obstructive uropathies that obstruct urine flow or prevent elimination are considered postrenal causes of ARF. If these conditions are corrected promptly, before renal parenchymal damage, complete recovery is possible.

Primary Nursing Diagnosis	**ALTERATION IN FLUID AND ELECTROLYTE BALANCE**
Definition	Disturbance in the amount of body fluid and disturbance in the values of body electrolytes
Possibly Related to	• Decreased renal perfusion • Renal parenchymal injury or disease • Obstruction of renal system
Characteristics	Oliguria Diuresis (early) Edema Hypertension Sudden weight gain Pruritis Fatigue Purpura Increased BUN Increased creatinine

Ascites
Hyperkalemia
  Arrhythmias
  Muscle weakness
  Peaking of T wave on EKG
  Intestinal colic
  Diarrhea
Hypocalcemia
  Arrhythmias
  Muscle cramps
  Tetany
  Seizures
Hyponatremia (dilutional)
  Seizures
  Muscle cramps/twitching
  Lethargy
  Weakness
  Coma
Metabolic acidosis

Expected Outcomes

Child will resume fluid and electrolyte balance as evidenced by

a. adequate urine output (state specific highest and lowest outputs for each child; normal, 1 to 2 ml/kg/hour
b. receipt of only the ordered amount of fluid intake (state exact amount allowed for each child)
c. blood pressure within acceptable range (state specific highest and lowest blood pressures for each child)
d. BUN between 5 and 18 mg/dl
e. creatinine between 0.3 and 1.0 mg/dl
f. lack of

—sudden weight gain
—pruritis
—fatigue

—purpura
—ascites

g. serum potassium between 3.5 and 5.0 mEq/liter
h. serum calcium between 8.8 and 10.8 mg/dl
i. serum sodium between 138 and 145 mEq/liter
j. serum carbon dioxide between 18 and 27 mEq/liter

Possible Nursing Interventions

- Keep accurate record of intake and output.
- If Foley catheter is in place, note hourly output. Maintain asceptic technique when emptying urine and caring for catheter.
- Assess and record

—signs/symptoms of alteration in fluid and electrolyte balance (such as those listed under "Characteristics") every 2 hours and PRN
—laboratory values as indicated. Report any abnormalities to the physician.
—blood pressure every 2 hours and PRN
—IV fluids and condition of IV site every hour

- Ensure that medications (calcium gluconate, sodium bicarbonate, glucose, insulin, kayexalate, Amphojel, and hydralazine) are administered on schedule if ordered. Assess and record effectiveness and any side effects.
- Weigh child daily (or as ordered) on same scale at the same time of day.

- Ensure that peritoneal dialysis is being done according to hospital policy, including

  —maintaining a closed sterile system
  —using aseptic technique whenever the sytem is opened
  —warming the dialysate
  —obtaining daily cultures
  —changing tubing and catheter site dressing every 24 hours using sterile technique

- Record child's response to peritoneal dialysis including untoward reactions such as fever, abdominal pain, and change in level of consciousness.

Evaluation for Charting

- State intake and output.
- Describe condition of IV site.
- State current laboratory values.
- State highest and lowest B/P.
- State child's weight and determine whether it has increased or decreased since the previous weighing.
- Describe any signs/symptoms of alteration in fluid and electrolyte balance (such as those listed under "Characteristics").
- State whether medications were administered on schedule. Describe effectiveness and any side effects.
- State whether peritoneal dialysis was used. If so, describe procedure and child's response.

ALTERATION IN PATTERNS OF URINARY ELIMINATION, RETENTION

Nursing Diagnosis

Definition Inability of the body to eliminate urine adequately

Possibly Related to	• Urinary tract anomalies
	• Obstructive uropathies
Characteristics	Oliguria
	Edema
	Hypertension
	Headache
	Sudden weight gain

Expected Outcomes

Child will be free of urinary retention as evidenced by

  a. adequate urinary output (state specific highest and lowest outputs for each child; normal, 1 to 2 ml/kg/hour)
  b. blood pressure within acceptable range (state specific highest and lowest B/P for each child)
  c. lack of

   —headache
   —edema

  d. return to preillness body weight

Possible Nursing Interventions

• Keep accurate record of intake and output. Be sure that child does not exceed maximal intake ordered.
• Assess and record

   —B/P every 2 hours and PRN
   —signs/symptoms of urinary retention (such as those listed under "Characteristics") every 2 hours and PRN

• Weigh child daily on same scale at the same time of day.

Evaluation for Charting

• State intake and output.
• Describe any signs/symptoms of urinary retention (such as those listed under "Characteristics").

- State highest and lowest B/P.
- State child's weight and determine whether it has increased or decreased since the previous weighing.

Related Nursing Diagnoses

DECREASED CARDIAC OUTPUT related to

a. circulatory congestion
b. hypertension

ALTERATION IN NUTRITION: LESS THAN BODY REQUIREMENTS related to increased tissue catabolism

POTENTIAL FOR INFECTION related to

a. invasive treatments/procedures
b. poor systemic perfusion
c. poor nutritional state

INEFFECTIVE FAMILY COPING related to the seriousness and emergency nature of the disease

HEMOLYTIC-UREMIC SYNDROME

Pathophysiology

Hemolytic-uremic syndrome (HUS) is a clinical condition of hemolytic anemia, thrombocytopenia, and acute renal failure. The cause of HUS remains unclear. There seem to be many stimuli (bacterial and viral agents, immunological responses, and genetics) that initiate the sequence of microangiopathic hemolytic anemia, increased platelet destruction, and impaired renal function.

Vascular endothelial damage is the main pathologic process of HUS, occurring in areas of high blood flow, such as the kidney. In the kidneys, the glomerular endothelial cells become swollen, separate from the glomerular basement membrane, and deposit themselves in the arterioles and capillaries. These endothelial cells, along with fibrin deposits, cause partial or complete obstruction of the renal arterioles and capillaries. As blood flows through these damaged and narrowed vessels, platelets and erythrocytes become fragmented and are then removed from circulation by the spleen, resulting in hemolytic anemia.

Thrombocytopenia in HUS occurs for several reasons. Platelets aggregate wherever there is vascular endothelial damage. Platelet aggregation also occurs because of nucleotide release from damaged red blood cells, and there is platelet destruction as damaged platelets are removed from circulation by the spleen. Acute renal failure occurs in HUS because of renal ischemia or necrosis caused by decreased blood flow to the kidneys and the decreased glomerular filtration rate.

HUS occurs most often in infants under 1 year of age or in children aged 3 to 7. Frequently there is a diarrheal or upper respiratory infection prodrome. Medical treatment is supportive and the child's prognosis correlates with the extent of glomerular damage.

Primary Nursing Diagnosis

FLUID VOLUME EXCESS

Definition

An increase in the amount of circulating fluid volume

Possibly Related to

- Decreased renal blood flow
- Decreased glomerular filtration rate

Characteristics

Oliguria or anuria
Hypervolemia
Blood pressure changes
Edema
Sudden weight gain
Hepatosplenomegaly
Proteinuria
Urinary cell casts
Abdominal pain
Lethargy
Irritability
Fever

Expected Outcomes

Child will resume fluid balance as evidenced by

a. adequate urine output (state specific highest and lowest outputs for each child; normal, 1 to 2 ml/kg/hour

b. blood pressure within acceptable range (state specific highest and

lowest blood pressures for each child)
c. clear, pale-yellow urine
d. temperature of 36.5° to 37.2° C
e. lack of

—proteinuria
—edema
—sudden weight gain
—abdominal pain
—hepatomegaly
—lethargy
—irritability

Possible Nursing Interventions

- Keep accurate record of intake and output. Be sure that child does not exceed maximal intake ordered. Document characteristics of urinary output.
- If Foley catheter is in place, keep hourly output. Maintain aseptic technique when emptying urine and administering catheter care.
- Assess and record

—signs/symptoms of fluid volume excess (such as those listed under "Characteristics") every 2 hours and PRN
—blood pressure and temperature every 2 hours and PRN
—IV fluids and condition of IV site every hour

- Weigh child BID on same scale at the same time of day.
- Ensure that peritoneal dialysis is being done according to hospital policy including

—maintaining a closed sterile system
—using aseptic technique whenever the system is opened
—warming dialysate

—obtaining daily cultures
—changing tubing and catheter site dressing every 24 hours using sterile technique

- Record child's response to peritoneal dialysis including untoward reactions such as fever, abdominal pain, and change in level of consciousness.
- Ensure that antihypertensives (hydralazine) and antipyretics are administered on schedule if ordered. Assess and record effectiveness and any side effects (such as nausea/vomiting, headache, and tachycardia).

Evaluation for Charting

- State intake and output.
- Describe characteristics of urine output.
- Describe any signs/symptoms of fluid volume excess (such as those listed under "Characteristics").
- Describe amount and location of edema.
- State highest and lowest temperature and B/P.
- State child's weight and determine whether it has increased or decreased since the previous weighing.
- State whether peritoneal dialysis was used. If so, describe procedure and child's response.
- State whether medications were administered on schedule. Describe effectiveness and any side effects.

ALTERATION IN TISSUE PERFUSION/OXYGENATION

Nursing Diagnosis

Definition Inadequate amount of blood and oxygen being delivered to the tissues in the body

Possibly Related to Characteristics

Damaged and destroyed blood cells
Purpura
Rectal bleeding
Bloody diarrhea
Decreased platelets
Decreased hematocrit/hemoglobin
Petechiae
Bruising
Distended abdomen
Tachycardia
Hematuria

Expected Outcomes

Child's tissue will have adequate supply of blood and oxygen as evidenced by

    a. hematocrit/hemoglobin within acceptable range (state specific range for each child)
    b. platelets between 150,000 and 400,000/mm^3
    c. heart rate within acceptable range (state specific highest and lowest rate for each child)
    d. lack of

       —purpura
       —rectal bleeding
       —bloody diarrhea
       —petechiae
       —bruising
       —abdominal distention
       —hematuria

Possible Nursing Interventions

• Assess and record

    —heart rate every 2 hours and PRN
    —laboratory values as indicated. Report abnormalities to the physician.
    —signs/symptoms of decreased tissue perfusion/oxygenation (such as

those listed under "Characteristics") every 2 hours and PRN
—abdominal girth every shift

- Transfuse blood products as ordered. Assess, record, and report any signs/symptoms of transfusion reaction (such as chills, fever, headache, flank pain, urticaria, bruising, chest pain, difficulty breathing, irregular heart rate, and apprehension).
- Guaiac test all stools, emesis, and nasogastric drainage. Record results.
- Handle child gently to prevent bruising.

Evaluation for Charting

- State highest and lowest heart rate.
- State current laboratory values and results of guaiac testing.
- Describe any signs/symptoms of decreased tissue perfusion/oxygenation (such as those listed under "Characteristics").
- State type and amount of any blood products transfused and state post-transfusion laboratory values. Describe any signs/symptoms of transfusion reaction.
- State current abdominal girth and determine whether it has increased or decreased since previous girth measurement.

Related Nursing Diagnoses

ELECTROLYTE IMBALANCE related to

a. decreased perfusion to kidneys
b. decreased glomerular filtration rate

DECREASED CARDIAC OUTPUT related to

a. fluid volume excess

    b. damaged or destroyed blood cells

ALTERATION IN LEVEL OF CON-
SCIOUSNESS related to electrolyte
imbalance

DISTURBANCE IN SELF-CON-
CEPT: BODY IMAGE related to

    a. edema

    b. sudden weight gain

    c. petechiae, purpura, and bruising

DIABETES INSIPIDUS

Pathophysiology
There are two types of diabetes insipidus. Neurogenic (central) diabetes insipidus results in hyposecretion of antidiuretic hormone (ADH) and can occur after head trauma or brain surgery or can be caused by incomplete formation of the pituitary gland. In nephrogenic diabetes insipidus the kidneys do not respond to ADH. This type of diabetes insipidus is an X-linked recessive genetic defect and does not respond to vasopressin administration.

ADH is produced in the hypothalamus. It is stored in and released from the posterior pituitary gland. Water is normally conserved in the body when the distal renal tubules respond to ADH stimulation. In diabetes insipidus there is either a lack of ADH (neurogenic) or decreased renal responsiveness to ADH (nephrogenic); therefore, the kidneys are unable to conserve water. As the osmolality of the plasma increases, interstitial and intracellular water is pulled into the intravascular space, resulting in diuresis and hypernatremia. The child experiences polyuria and polydipsia. If the child cannot maintain adequate fluid intake, significant dehydration can occur. Severe hypernatremia accompanied by dehydration can result in seizures, coma, and death.

**Primary Nursing
Diagnosis**

FLUID VOLUME DEFICIT

Definition
A decrease in the amount of circulating fluid volume

Possibly Related to Polyuria secondary to

- lack of ADH
- decreased responsiveness of the kidneys to ADH

Characteristics Polyuria

Polydipsia

Urine specific gravity of less than 1.005

Decreased urine osmolality (less than 200 mOsm/liter)

Increased serum sodium (greater than 145 mEq/liter)

Increased serum osmolality (greater than 300 mOsm/kg)

Enuresis

Decreased urine sodium (less than 130 mEq/24 hours

Intense thirst for water

Dry mucous membranes

Poor skin turgor

Weight loss

Irritability

Tachycardia, hypotension

Sunken fontanel

Cool extremities

Prolonged capillary refill, longer than 2 to 3 seconds

Weak peripheral pulses

Expected Outcomes Child will have an adequate fluid volume as evidenced by

a. adequate fluid intake, IV or oral (state exact amount of intake needed for each child)
b. adequate urinary output (state specific highest and lowest outputs for each child; normal, 1 to 2 ml/kg/hour
c. Urine specific gravity of 1.008 to 1.020

d. Urine osmolality of 500 to 800 mOsm/liter
e. Serum osmolality of 280 to 295 mOsm/kg
f. serum sodium of 138 to 145 mEq/liter
g. urine sodium of 130 to 200 mEq/24 hours
h. moist mucous membranes
i. rapid skin recoil
j. heart rate and blood pressure within acceptable range (state specific highest and lowest parameters for each child)
k. lack of signs/symptoms of fluid volume deficit (such as those listed under "Characteristics")

Possible Nursing Interventions

- Keep accurate record of intake and output.
- Assess and record

  —IV fluid and condition of IV site every hour
  —signs/symptoms of fluid volume deficit (such as those listed under "Characteristics") every 2 hours and PRN
  —heart rate and B/P every 2 hours and PRN
  —laboratory values as indicated. Report abnormalities to the physician.
  —daily weight.

- Check and record urine specific gravity every void or as ordered.
- Assist with water deprivation testing.
- Ensure that vasopressin is administered by the prescribed route. Assess and record effectiveness and any side

effects (such as abdominal cramping and tachycardia/bradycardia).

Evaluation for Charting

- State intake and output.
- Describe condition of IV site.
- Describe status of mucous membranes and skin turgor.
- Describe any signs/symptoms of fluid volume deficit (such as those listed under "Characteristics").
- State highest and lowest heart rates and B/P.
- State highest and lowest urine specific gravity values.
- State weight and indicate whether it has increased or decreased since previous weighing.
- State whether vasopressin was given on schedule. Describe effectiveness and any side effects.
- Describe any therapeutic measures used to maintain adequate fluid volume and their effectiveness.

ALTERATION IN ELECTROLYTE BALANCE: SODIUM EXCESS

Nursing Diagnosis

Definition

A disturbance in the value of the body's sodium

Possibly Related to

Polyuria secondary to lack of ADH or unresponsiveness of kidney to ADH

Characteristics

Hypernatremia
Lethargy
Seizures
Coma
Dry mucous membranes
Flushed skin
Intense thirst
Serum osmolality

Expected Outcomes

Child will have adequate sodium balance as evidenced by

a. serum sodium between 138 and 145 mEq/liter
b. appropriate level of consciousness for age
c. serum osmolality between 280 and 295 mOsm/kg
d. lack of signs/symptoms of sodium excess (such as those listed under "Characteristics").

Possible Nursing Interventions

• Assess and record

—neurologic vital signs every 2 hours and PRN
—laboratory values as indicated. Report abnormalities to the physician.
—signs/symptoms of sodium excess (such as those listed under "Characteristics") every 2 hours and PRN

• Keep accurate record of intake and output.

Evaluation for Charting

• Describe child's neurological status.
• State current laboratory values.
• Describe any signs/symptoms of sodium excess (such as those listed under "Characteristics").
• State intake and output.
• Describe any therapeutic measures used to correct sodium excess and their effectiveness.

Related Nursing Diagnoses

ALTERATION IN LEVEL OF CONSCIOUSNESS related to hypernatremia

DECREASED CARDIAC OUTPUT related to severe fluid volume deficit

ALTERATION IN PATTERNS OF URINARY ELIMINATION related to lack of ADH or unresponsiveness of kidneys to ADH

INEFFECTIVE FAMILY COPING related to

a. underlying disease state
b. genetic nature of illness
c. knowledge deficit

Medical Diagnosis

DIABETIC KETOACIDOSIS

Pathophysiology

Diabetic ketoacidosis is a catabolic state resulting from insulin insufficiency. Insulin is necessary for the body to facilitate the entrance of intravascular glucose into muscle and fat cells, store glucose (as glycogen) in the liver and muscle cells, and prevent fat mobilization. When there is a lack of insulin these activities are impaired, leading to hyperglycemia, dehydration, and ketoacidosis.

With insufficient insulin, hyperglycemia occurs because intravascular glucose is unable to enter the cells. As a result glycogen is broken down in the liver as gluconeogenesis is stimulated. This hyperglycemia contributes to osmotic diuresis, which causes water loss, electrolyte imbalance, and eventually dehydration.

Most cells require glucose as their primary energy source. When glucose is unable to enter the cells, another energy source is used, principally free fatty acids released from adipose tissue. Ketone bodies are the end product of fatty acid metabolism. The substantial accumulation of these ketone bodies alters the serum pH, resulting in ketoacidosis. Coma and death may occur with severe hyperglycemia or ketoacidosis.

The treatment goals for a child with diabetic ketoacidosis include the administration of effective doses of insulin, correction of fluid volume deficit, correction of serum electrolyte imbalance and acid-base imbalance, and the prevention of complications (such as renal failure or cerebral edema).

Primary Nursing Diagnosis

ALTERATION IN METABOLIC FUNCTION

Definition

Imbalance in the body of the utilization of specific biochemicals

Possibly Related to

- Unstable blood glucose levels
- Insufficient insulin
- Increased insulin requirements secondary to infection, illness, or stress

Characteristics

Hyperglycemia (greater than 300 mg/dl)
Dehydration
Metabolic acidosis, pH less than 7.4
Polyuria
Polydipsia
Acetone breath
Polyphagia or anorexia
Kussmaul breathing
EKG changes
Electrolyte imbalance
Headache, lethargy, confusion, irritability
Decreased visual acuity, blurred vision
Glysouria
Acetone in urine
Nausea and vomiting
Abdominal pain
Coma

Expected Outcomes

Child will have adequate metabolic function as evidenced by

a. stable serum glucose level between 60 and 180 mg/dl
b. lack of

—signs/symptoms of hyperglycemia (e.g., lethargy, polydipsia, polyuria, dehydration, nausea and vomiting, abdominal pain, cetone breath, Kussmaul breathing, glycosuria, and ketonuria)

—signs/symptoms of hypoglycemia (e.g., irritability, headache, polyphagia, impaired vision)

c. normal sinus rhythm
d. serum pH of 7.35 to 7.45
e. aceptable range for serum electrolytes (state specific range for each child)

Possible Nursing Interventions

• Assess and record

—blood glucose levels every 2 hours and PRN (serum, Chemstrip, glucometer)

—serum electrolyte and pH values as indicated

—signs/symptoms of hyperglycemia or hypoglycemia (such as those listed under "Characteristics") every 2 hours and PRN

—insulin drip (usual initial dose, 0.1 unit/kg/hour) every hour along with the condition of the IV site. Use a separate line for IV insulin administration. Change tubing according to hospital policy. Discontinue insulin drip approximately 30 minutes after initial subcutaneous dose if ordered.

• Place child on cardiac monitor while administering IV insulin. Notify physician of any abnormalities.

• Evaluate and record results of EKG strips at least once/shift.

• Keep accurate record of intake and output.

- Maintain bedside diabetic flow sheet to include blood glucose levels, insulin dose, and urine testing results.
- Administer oxygen in the correct amount and by the correct route if ordered. Assess and record the effectiveness of therapy.

Evaluation for Charting

- State highest and lowest blood glucose levels and urine testing results.
- State highest and lowest serum pH and electrolyte values.
- Describe any signs/symptoms of hyperglycemia or hypoglycemia (such as those listed under "Characteristics").
- State intake and output.
- Describe condition of IV site. State rate and IV insulin dosage.
- Document EKG interpretation.
- Describe any therapeutic measures used to correct diabetic ketoacidosis and their effectiveness.

Nursing Diagnosis

FLUID VOLUME DEFICIT

Definition

A decrease in the amount of circulating fluid volume

Possibly Related to

- Osmotic diuresis secondary to hyperglycemia
- Vomiting

Characteristics

Flushed dry skin
Polyuria, nocturia
Vomiting, nausea
Kussmaul breathing
Dry mucous membranes
Poor skin turgor
Weight loss
Tachycardia, hypotension

Expected Outcomes

Child will have an adequate fluid volume as evidenced by

    a. adequate fluid intake, IV or oral (state exact amount of intake needed for each child)

    b. adequate urinary output (sate specific highest and lowest outputs for each child; normal, 1 to 2 ml/kg/hour

    c. moist mucous membranes

    d. rapid skin recoil

    e. lack of weight loss

    f. heart rate and blood pressure within acceptable range (state specific highest and lowest parameters for each child)

Possible Nursing Interventions

- Keep accurate record of intake and output. Keep hourly output if foley catheter is in place.
- Assess and record

  —IV fluid and condition of IV site every hour. Fluid losses through urine and GI tract may need to be replaced by IV fluids.

  —signs/symptoms of fluid volume deficit (such as those listed under "Characteristics") every 2 hours and PRN

  —heart rate and B/P every 2 hours and PRN.

- Give mouth care every 4 hours and PRN.
- Record daily weight.
- Administer volume expanders (such as 5% albumin) as ordered if shock is present.

Evaluation for Charting

- State intake and output.

- Describe condition of IV site and state type of IV fluids in use.
- Describe status of mucous membranes and skin turgor.
- State highest and lowest heart rate and B/P.
- State weight and indicate whether it has increased or decreased since previous weighing.
- Describe any therapeutic measures used to maintain adequate fluid volume and their effectiveness.

ALTERATION IN ELECTROLYTE BALANCE: SODIUM AND POTASSIUM

Nursing Diagnosis

Definition

A disturbance in the value of the body's sodium and potassium

Possibly Related to

Sodium losses secondary to vomiting and osmotic diuresis

Temporary increased extracellular potassium (false high) secondary to

—acidosis
—insulin deficiency
—dehydration

- Potassium losses secondary to

—polyuria
—insulin administration
—dilution resulting from rehydration
—correction of acidosis (potassium reenters the cells)

Characteristics

Hyponatremia
Weakness
Delirium
Hyperkalemia (false high)
EKG changes: spiked T wave, widened QRS complex, flattened P wave, and ectopic beats

Weakness
Flushed skin
Hypokalemia
  EKG changes: flat T wave, peaked P
  wave, ectopic beats
  Hypotension and rapid pulse
  Coma

Expected Outcomes

Child will have adequate electrolyte balance as evidenced by

a. serum sodium between 138 and 145 mEq/liter
b. serum potassium between 3.5 and 5.0 mEq/liter
c. normal sinus rhythm and EKG configuration
d. lack of signs/symptoms of electrolyte imbalance (such as those listed under "Characteristics").

Possible Nursing Interventions

- Assess and record heart rate and B/P every 2 hours and PRN.
- Keep accurate record of intake and output.
- Assess and record any signs/symptoms of electrolyte imbalance (such as those listed under "Characteristics") every 2 hours and PRN. Report any abnormalities to the physician.
- Ensure that proper electrolyte supplements are added to the IV fluids.
- Evaluate and record results of EKG strips at least once/shift.
- Assess and record laboratory values as indicated. Report abnormalities to the physician.

Evaluation for Charting

- State highest and lowest heart rate and B/P.
- State intake and output.

- Describe any signs/symptoms of electrolyte imbalance (such as those listed under "Characteristics").
- Document EKG interpretation.
- Describe any therapeutic measures used to correct electrolyte imbalance and their effectiveness.
- State current laboratory values.

Related Nursing Diagnoses

ALTERATION IN LEVEL OF CONSCIOUSNESS related to cerebral edema

ALTERATION IN NUTRITION: LESS THAN BODY REQUIREMENTS related to

a. decreased appetite
b. unstable blood glucose levels

INEFFECTIVE FAMILY COPING related to

a. long-term illness and prognosis
b. need for continual monitoring of blood glucose, urine acetone, and diet on a daily basis

SYNDROME OF INAPPROPRIATE SECRETION OF ANTIDIURETIC HORMONE (SIADH)

Pathophysiology

Normally, antidiuretic hormone (ADH) is released from the posterior pituitary gland in response to increased serum osmotic pressure or hypovolemia. The syndrome of inappropriate secretion of antidiuretic hormone (SIADH) is the excessive or inappropriate release of antidiuretic hormone. This inappropriate or excessive secretion of ADH results in increased reabsorption of water from the renal tubules causing intravascular fluid overload, which may then shift into the intracellular space. Subsequently, hyponatremia occurs.

SIADH is seen most often in children with central nervous system disorders such as bacterial meningitis, encephalitis, head trauma, and Guillain-Barré syndrome. It may also occur with a variety of other disorders (i.e., tuberculosis, cirrhosis, or pancreatic carcinoma or after mitral valve repair).

Primary Nursing Diagnosis

ALTERATION IN ELECTROLYTE BALANCE: SODIUM LOSSES

Definition

A disturbance in the value of the body's sodium

Possibly Related to

Increased intravascular fluid secondary to inappropriate ADH secretion

Characteristics

Hyponatremia
Oliguria (less than one ml/kg/hour)
Weakness
Delirium

Seizures
Lethargy
Stupor
Coma
Headache
Anorexia
Nausea/vomiting
Confusion
Muscle twitching
Decreased deep tendon reflexes
Positive Babinski reflex

Expected Outcomes

Child will have adequate sodium balance as evidenced by:

a. serum sodium between 138 and 145 mEq/liter
b. adequate urine output (state specific highest and lowest outputs for each child; normal, 1 to 2 ml/kg/hour
c. appropriate level of consciousness for age
d. lack of signs/symptoms of decreased serum sodium levels (such as those listed under "Characteristics")

Possible Nursing Interventions

- Assess and record

    —neurologic vital signs every 2 hours and PRN
    —laboratory values as indicated. Report abnormalities to the physician.
    —signs/symptoms of decreased serum sodium (such as those listed under "Characteristics") every 2 hours and PRN

- Keep accurate record of intake and output.

- Administer 3% saline solution with potassium supplements and IV Lasix (furosemide) if ordered. Assess and record urine sodium and potassium concentrations to determine therapeutic effectiveness.

Evaluation for Charting

- Describe child's neurologic status.
- State current laboratory values.
- Describe any signs/symptoms of decreased serum sodium (such as those listed under "Characteristics").
- Describe any therapeutic measures used to increase serum sodium levels and their effectiveness.
- State intake and output.

FLUID VOLUME EXCESS (INTRAVASCULAR)

Nursing Diagnosis

Definition Increased circulating fluid volume in the body

Possibly Related to Increased water reabsorption from renal tubules secondary to inappropriate ADH secretion

Characteristics Hyponatremia

Serum hypoosmolality (less than 270 mOsm/kg)

Hypotonicity

Increased urine sodium

Urine specific gravity greater than 1.012

Inappropriately increased urine osmolality as compared to serum osmolality

Sudden weight gain

Expected Outcomes Child will resume fluid balance as evidenced by

a. serum sodium of 138 to 145 mEq/ liter

b. urine osmolality of 500 to 800 mOsm/liter (usually about 1.5 to 3 times greater than serum osmolality)

c. serum osmolality of 280 to 295 mOsm/kg

d. urine sodium of 130 to 200 mEq/ 24 hours

e. urine specific gravity of 1.008 to 1.020

f. lack of sudden weight gain

Possible Nursing Interventions

- Keep accurate record of intake and output. Restrict fluid intake as ordered (the degree of hypoosmolality and hyponatremia will determine the amount of fluid restriction).
- Assess and record

  —IV fluid and condition of IV site every hour.

  —laboratory values as indicated. Report abnormalities to the physician.

  —signs/symptoms of fluid volume excess (such as those listed under "Characteristics") every 2 hours and PRN

- Record daily weight.
- Check and record urine specific gravity every void or as ordered.

Evaluation for Charting

- State intake and output.
- Describe condition of IV site.
- State current laboratory values.
- Describe any signs/symptoms of fluid volume excess (such as those listed under "Characteristics").
- State weight and indicate whether it has increased or decreased since previous weighing.

- State highest and lowest urine specific gravity values.

Related Nursing Diagnoses

ALTERATION IN LEVEL OF CONSCIOUSNESS related to cerebral edema secondary to hyponatremia resulting from increased intracellular fluid

ALTERATION IN PATTERNS OF URINARY ELIMINATION related to inappropriate ADH secretion

INEFFECTIVE CHILD AND FAMILY COPING related to underlying disease process

PARENTAL AND CHILD KNOWLEDGE DEFICIT related to

a. underlying disease process
b. treatments and procedures

Medical
Diagnosis
DISSEMINATED INTRAVASCULAR COAGULATION

Pathophysiology

Disseminated intravascular coagulation (DIC) is a complex physiologic process in which the body's hemostatic mechanism is disrupted. DIC is not a primary disorder, but occurs secondary to many major pathological processes, such as septic shock, burns, anoxia, trauma, surgery, and transfusion reactions.

The pathologic events that can trigger DIC include the circulation of endotoxins or antigen-antibody complexes; an increase in circulating coagulation factors; the presence of damaged red blood cells, platelets, or endothelial cells in the circulation; blood stasis; and the destruction of blood vessel walls.

DIC is characterized by coagulation followed by hemorrhage. The coagulation system is stimulated by a pathologic event and large amounts of thrombin are generated. Thrombin breaks down fibrinogen in to fibrin. Thrombin also causes platelet aggregation and platelet destruction, resulting in thrombocytopenia. Hemolytic anemia occurs as microthrombi deposit themselves in the capillaries and small vessels, damaging circulating red blood cells. Fibrinolysis is also stimulated by thrombin, resulting in hemorrhage as the clots dissolve.

Primary Nursing Diagnosis	**ALTERATION IN TISSUE PERFUSION/ OXYGENATION**
Definition	Inadequate amount of blood and oxygen being delivered to the tissues in the body
Possibly Related to	• Excessive coagulation • Fibrinolytic process
Characteristics	Petechiae Bruising Hematuria Epistaxis Hemoptysis GI bleeding Gingival bleeding Oozing or diffuse bleeding from puncture sites Decreased platelets Prolonged PT and PTT Decreased hemoglobin and hematocrit Hypotension Phlebitis Acrocyanosis
Expected Outcomes	Child's tissue will have adequate supply of blood and oxygen as evidenced by

a. hemoglobin/hematocrit within acceptable range (state specific range for each child)
b. platelets between 150,000 and 400,000/mm^3
c. PT within acceptable range of 11 to 16 seconds (normal values will be set by each laboratory)
d. PTT within acceptable range of 30 to 45 seconds
e. blood pressure within acceptable range (state specific highest and lowest blood pressures for each child)

f. lack of

—petechiae
—bruising
—phlebitis
—acrocyanosis

Possible Nursing Interventions

- Assess and record

  —B/P every 2 hours and PRN
  —laboratory values as indicated. Report abnormalities to the physician.
  —signs/symptoms of decreased tissue perfusion/oxygenation (such as those listed under ("Characteristics") every 2 hours and PRN

- Transfuse blood products as ordered. Assess, record, and report any signs/symptoms of transfusion reaction (such as chills, fever, headache, flank pain, urticaria, bruising, chest pain, difficulty breathing, irregular heart rate, and apprehension).
- Handle child gently to prevent bleeding and bruising.
- Guaiac test all stools, emesis, and nasogastric drainage. Record results.
- Ensure that heparin is being administered as ordered. Assess and record effectiveness and any side efffects (such as flushing, sudden hypotension, bradycardia, and dyspnea).
- Apply pressure dressings as indicated to puncture sites.

Evaluation for Charting

- State highest and lowest B/P.
- State current laboratory values and results of guaiac testing.
- Describe any signs/symptoms of decreased tissue perfusion/oxygenation.

- State type and amount of any blood products transfused and state post-transfusion laboratory values. Describe any signs/symptoms of transfusion reaction.
- State whether heparin was administered as ordered. Describe effectiveness and any side effects.
- Describe any therapeutic measures used to enhance tissue perfusion/oxygenation and their effectiveness.

Nursing Diagnosis

DECREASED CARDIAC OUTPUT

Definition

A decrease in the amount of blood that leaves the left ventricle

Possibly Related to

- Hemorrhage secondary to fibrinolysis
- Decreased tissue perfusion/oxgenation

Characteristics

Tachycardia

Hypotension

Decreased hematocrit and hemoglobin

Unequal, decreased, or absent peripheral pulses

Prolonged capillary refill, longer than 2 to 3 seconds

Cool, pale skin

Expected Outcomes

Child will maintain an adequate cardiac output as evidenced by

a. heart rate within acceptable range (state specific highest and lowest rates for each child)

b. blood pressure within acceptable range (state specific highest and lowest blood pressures for each child)

c. hematocrit/hemoglobin within acceptable range (state specific range for each child)

d. strong and equal peripheral pulses
e. brisk capillary refill, within 2 and 3 seconds
f. skin warm to touch
g. lack of paleness

Possible Nursing Interventions

• Assess and record

—apical rate and blood pressure every 1 to 2 hours and PRN
—laboratory values as indicated. Report abnormalities to the physician.
—signs/symptoms of decreased cardiac output (such as those listed under "Characteristics") every 2 hours and PRN

• Transfuse blood products as ordered. Assess, record, and report any signs/symptoms of transfusion reaction (such as chills, fever, headache, flank pain, urticaria, bruising, chest pain, difficulty breathing, irregular heart rate, and apprehension).
• Evaluate and record results of EKG strips at least once/shift.
• Keep accurate record of intake and output.

Evaluation for Charting

• State highest and lowest apical rates and B/P.
• State current laboratory values.
• Describe any signs/symptoms of decreased cardiac output (such as those listed under "Characteristics").
• State type and amount of any blood products transfused and state post-transfusion laboratory values. Describe any signs/symptoms of transfusion reaction.

- Document EKG interpretation.
- State intake and output.

Related Nursing Diagnoses

IMPAIRED GAS EXCHANGE related to hypoxemia

ALTERATION IN LEVEL OF CONSCIOUSNESS related to alteration in tissue perfusion/oxygenation

FLUID VOLUME DEFICIT related to

a. hemorrhage
b. shock

CHILD/PARENTAL FEAR related to seriousness of illness

Medical Diagnosis

ACQUIRED IMMUNE DEFICIENCY SYNDROME

Pathophysiology

A child with acquired immune deficiency syndrome (AIDS) has been infected with the human immunodeficiency virus (HIV) and subsequently develops a cellular immunodeficiency. Other causes of immunodeficiencies in children (such as congenital immunodeficiencies and malignancies) should be excluded before a definitive diagnosis of AIDS is made.

The HIV is a retrovirus that causes an immune deficiency resulting in a decrease of cell-mediated immunity, rendering the child susceptible to numerous opportunistic infections and rare neoplasms. Once HIV enters the child's bloodstream, it becomes attached to a part of the T4 lymphocyte and enters the cells. Then, with the aid of the reverse transcriptase enzyme, DNA is produced from RNA. This DNA will produce new viral RNA, which can result in cellular death and produce viral particles leading to the spread of the HIV infection.

T cells are involved in the mediation of cellular immunity and in the regulation of B cell function, controlling B cell antibody responses to new antigens. The characteristics of HIV are that it selectively infects and destroys T4 lymphocytes. Macrophages and neural cells can also be infected. Pediatric AIDS patients experience a decrease in the number of helper T cells and a reversal of the helper to suppressor T cell ratio, resulting in depression of the child's cellular immunity. This leads to infections with opportunistic agents. The loss of T cell regulation of B cell function leaves the AIDS child unable to respond properly to new antigens, making the child particularly vulnerable to common bacterial infections. These infections can become recurrent and life-threatening. Examples include pneumonia, meningitis, and sepsis. Causative organisms include *Haemophilus influenzae*, *Staphylococcus aureus*, *Staphylococcus epidermidis*, *Streptococcus pneumoniae*, *Streptococcus pyogenes*, and some gram-negative enteric bacteria.

HIV infection can cause a wide spectrum of clinical manifestations varying from no symptoms to severe opportunistic infections, neurological deterioration, pulmonary failures, or death. Most children with AIDS present with a triad of failure to thrive, hepatosplenomegaly, and chronic interstitial pneumonitis. Because the lack of a cellular immune response, many children present with two or more opportunistic infections. The three most common opportunistic infections that occur with pediatric AIDS are *Pneumocystis carinii* pneumonia, invasive candidal esophagitis, and disseminated cytomegalovirus.

The majority of pediatric AIDS patients acquire the infection during the perinatal period and have mothers who have AIDS or are at an increased risk to develop AIDS. Many of these children have at least one parent who is an intravenous drug user. A small portion of pediatric AIDS cases are associated with blood or blood product transfusions. These include children with coagulation disorders and infants who received transfusions during the neonatal period.

The development of life-threatening infections usually requires that the pediatric AIDS patient be admitted to the critical care unit. The goals for treatment are to treat the infection, to support the involved systems, and to provide psychological support. The pediatric AIDS patient's short-term prognosis depends largely on the nature of the infectious agents involved and the degree of immunocompromise.

Primary Nursing Diagnosis	**ACTUAL INFECTION AND POTENTIAL FOR FURTHER INFECTION**
Definition	A condition in which the body is invaded by microorganisms
Possibly Related to	• Acquired cellular immunodeficiency • Opportunistic agents • Common bacterial agents
Characteristics	Fever/hypothermia Malaise Fatigue Night sweats Enlarged lymph nodes Skin rashes and mucous membrane lesions Change in level of consciousness/meningeal signs Diarrhea Cough Dyspnea Altered completed blood count
Expected Outcomes	Child will be free of secondary infection as evidenced by

a. body temperature within acceptable range of 36.5° to 37.2° C
b. clear and intact skin and mucous membranes
c. alertness when awake
d. orientation ×3 (if age-appropriate)
e. lack of signs/symptoms of infection (such as those listed under "Characteristics")
f. complete blood cell count within acceptable range (state specific highest and lowest counts for each child)

Possible Nursing Interventions

• Assess and record every 1 to 2 hours and PRN

—temperature
—signs/symptoms of infections (such as those listed under "Characteristics")

• Maintain good handwashing technique.
• Adhere to CDC guidlines and/or hospital policy for current isolation techniques.
• Obtain culture specimens (wound, blood, stool, sputum) if ordered. Label properly. Check results and notify physician of any abnormalities.
• Check and record results of CBC. Notify physician if CBC results are out of the acceptable range.
• Utilize tepid baths and cooling/heating blankets as indicated.
• Ensure that antibiotics, antiviral agents, antifungal agents, antipyretics, and gamma-globulin are administered on schedule. Assess and record effectiveness and any side effects.

Evaluation for Charting

- State highest and lowest temperature.
- Describe any signs/symptoms of infection (such as those listed under "Characteristics").
- Document isolation techniques utilized.
- State results of any cultures and/or CBC if available.
- State whether medications were administered on schedule. Describe effectiveness and any side effects.
- Describe any therapeutic measures used to treat the infection and make the child comfortable.

Nursing Diagnosis

IMPAIRED GAS EXCHANGE

Definition

Alteration in the exchange of oxygen and carbon dioxide in the lungs and/or at the cellular level

Possibly Related to

Invasion of the respiratory tract by microorganisms

Characteristics

Shortness of breath

Dyspnea

Cough

Tachypnea

Abnormal breath sounds (wheezes, rhonchi, crackles)

Cyanosis

Hypoxemia

Chest x-ray revealing interstitial infiltrates, pleural effusion, and/or pneumothorax

Retractions

Respiratory alkalosis or respiratory acidosis

Fatigue

Expected Outcomes Child will maintain adequate gas exchange as evidenced by

  a. respiratory rate within acceptable range (state highest and lowest rates for each child)
  b. clear and equal breath sounds bilaterally
  c. arterial pH of 7.35 to 7.45
  d. PaCO2 of 35 to 45 mm Hg
  e. PaO2 of 75 to 100 mm Hg
  h. arterial bicarbonate level of 22 to 28 mEq/liter
  i. clear chest x-ray
  j. lack of signs/symptoms of impaired gas exchange (such as those listed under "Characteristics")

Possible Nursing Interventions

• Assess and record every 1 to 2 hours and PRN

  —respiratory rate
  —breath sounds
  —color
  —signs/symptoms of impaired gas exchange (such as those listed under "Characteristics")

• Assess and record arterial blood gas values as ordered. Notify physician of any abnormalities.
• Administer humidified oxygen in the correct amount and by the correct route. Assess and record effectiveness of therapy.
• Suction using sterile technique every 2 hours and PRN. Record amount and characteristics of secretions.
• Ensure that chest physiotherapy is being done effectively and on schedule.

- If child is intubated, check ventilator settings (FiO2, Rate, PIP or TV, PEEP/CPAP) every 15 minutes. Record every 1 to 2 hours.
- Elevate head of bed to a 30° angle.
- Ensure that antibiotics and corticosteroids are administered on schedule. Assess and record effectiveness and any side effects.
- Check and record results of chest x-ray when indicated.

Evaluation for Charting

- State highest and lowest respiratory rate.
- Describe breath sounds.
- Describe any signs/symptoms of impaired gas exchange (such as those listed under "Characteristics").
- State highest and lowest arterial blood gas values and state the ongoing physiologic process (i.e., respiratory acidosis).
- State amount and route of oxygen delivery. Describe effectiveness.
- State type of endotracheal tube used and ventilator settings.
- State frequency of suctioning and describe amount and characteristics of secretions.
- State whether chest physiotherapy was done on schedule. Describe child's response to chest physiotherapy and its effectiveness in improving gas exchange.
- State results of chest x-ray if available.
- State whether head of bed was elevated.
- State whether antibiotics and/or corticosteroids were administered on

schedule. Describe effectiveness and any side effects.

ALTERATION IN NUTRITION: LESS THAN BODY REQUIREMENTS

Nursing Diagnosis

Definition Nutrients insufficient to meet body requirements

Possibly Related to

- Increased metabolic demands secondary to fever, increased respiratory rate, and sepsis
- Nausea and vomiting secondary to side effects of medications
- Diarrhea secondary to gram-negative enteric microorganisms
- Decreased oral intake secondary to painful oral lesions and inflamed esophagus

Characteristics Anorexia
Weight loss/failure to gain weight
Vomiting
Diarrhea
Abdominal cramping
Muscle wasting
Dysphagia

Expected Outcomes Child will be adequately nourished as evidenced by

a. absorbing adequate amount of calories, parenterally and orally (state specific amount for each child)
b. steady weight gain
c. lack of

—vomiting
—diarrhea
—abdominal cramping
—muscle wasting
—dysphagia

Possible Nursing Interventions

- Keep accurate record of intake and output.
- Assess and record any signs/symptoms of alteration in nutrition (such as those listed under "Characteristics").
- Weigh child daily on same scale at same time of day.
- Maintain and record daily calorie count as indicated.
- Encourage child to eat by assessing likes/dislikes and, when possible, providing foods that child likes to eat.
- Offer small frequent feedings (six small meals/day).
- Administer tube feedings on schedule if indicated. Follow hospital policy for changing and care of the feeding tube.
- Administer total parenteral nutrition and intralipids when ordered. Follow hospital policy for maintenance of total parenteral nutrition (TPN) and intralipid line and monitoring and recording of serum gucose and lipid levels.
- Organize care to conserve energy.
- Ensure that antiemetics, antidiarrheals, and oral topical anesthetics are administered on schedule. Assess and record effectiveness and any side effects.

Evaluation for Charting

- State intake and output.
- Describe any signs/symptoms of alteration in nutrition (such as those listed under "Characteristics").
- State current weight and determine whether it has increased or decreased from previous weight.
- State caloric intake.

- Describe any therapeutic measures used to maintain adequate nutrition and their effectiveness.
- State whether medications were administered on schedule. Describe effectiveness and any side effects.

KNOWLEDGE DEFICIT, CHILD/PARENTAL/FAMILY

Nursing Diagnosis

Definition Lack of information concerning the child's disease and care

Possibly Related to

- Sensory overload (too much to learn all at once)
- Fear of emotional involvement with infant/child who will die
- Cognitive or cultural-language limitations
- Guilt of transmitting AIDS to the child
- Fear of contracting AIDS or spreading it to others
- Misconceptions or inaccurate information

Characteristics Verbalization by child/parents/family indicating lack of knowledge

Relation of incorrect information to members of the health care team

Inability to repeat correctly and comprehend information taught

Inability to demonstrate previously taught skills correctly

Inappropriate or hostile behavior

Expected Outcomes Child/parents/family will have an adequate knowledge base concerning disease state and care as evidenced by

a. ability to state information correctly
b. ability to demonstrate skills correctly

c. lack of inappropriate or hostile behavior

Possible Nursing Interventions

- Listen to the concerns and fears of the child/parents/family.
- Give correct information and literature to child/parent/family. Teach at appropriate level.
- Correct any incorrect information.
- Assist and observe child/parents/family in performing skills that have been taught. Record their ability to perform skills.
- Assign primary nurse as usual spokesperson to provide consistency.

Evaluation for Charting

- State whether child/parents/family verbalized a knowledge deficit.
- Note whether child/parents/family were able to restate taught information correctly
- State whether child/parents/family were able to perform skills previously taught. Describe ability.
- Describe any inappropriate or hostile behavior.

Related Nursing Diagnoses

INEFFECTIVE FAMILY COPING related to

a. severity and nature of illness
b. poor prognosis

FEAR, CHILD/PARENT related to

a. severity and nature of illness
b. contraction from or spread of disease to others
c. death

BURNS, MAJOR THERMAL INJURY

Pathophysiology

Burns are a common cause of accidental injury in children. The causes of burns include thermal, electrical, chemical and radioactive agents.

Superficial (first degree) burns involve damage to the epidermis resulting in redness, edema, and pain, but no blistering. Partial-thickness (second degree) burns involve damage to both the epidermis and a portion of the dermis, resulting in a cherry red to glassy white appearance, edema, blister formation, exudate, pain, and possible damage to cutaneous nerve endings. With both of these types of burns, capillaries are usually intact, permitting tissue blanching and refill. Hair follicles, sebaceous glands, sweat glands, and some protective functions may also remain intact. Systemic effects range from minimal to severe. Superficial and most partial-thickness burns are usually able to heal by reepithelialization, especially if they are protected from further injury and infection. Deep partial-thickness burns may require autografting.

Full-thickness (third degree) burns involve destruction of all skin layers. As a result, hair follicles, sweat glands, sebaceous glands, and nerves are also destroyed. These burns vary in appearance from pearly white, tan, and brown to mahogany or black. They typically are not painful and blisters are not present. There is no blanching or refill. The term eschar is used to refer to the burned tissue of a full-thickness burn.

Skin grafting will be needed to close these wounds as regeneration of the skin is not possible once the dermis and dermal structures are destroyed. Full-thickness burns may also involve damage to fat, muscle, and bones.

Along with local pathologic changes, burns involve alterations in numerous organ systems as they respond to the injury. There can be various pulmonary problems, fluid and electrolyte shifts, sepsis, cardiovascular changes, extensive metabolic changes, acute renal failure, gastrointestinal involvement, and central nervous system dysfunction.

Primary Nursing Diagnosis

FLUID VOLUME DEFICIT

Definition

A decrease in the amount of circulating fluid volume

Possibly Related to

- Fluid loss from burn wound
- Shift of plasma to interstitium

Characteristics

Edema
Decreased urinary output
Decreased CVP/hypovolemia
Tachycardia
Hypotension
Confusion
Restlessness
Increased urine specific gravity
Dry mucous membranes

Expected Outcomes

Child will have an adequate fluid volume as evidenced by

a. lack of edema
b. adequate urinary output (state specific highest and lowest output for each child; normal, 1 to 2 ml/kg/hour

c. adequate IV fluid intake (state exact amount of intake needed for each child)
d. CVP between 4 and 8 mm Hg
e. heart rate and blood pressure within acceptable range (state specific highest and lowest parameters for each child)
f. lack of confusion
g. lack of extreme restlessness
h. urine specific gravity of 1.008 to 1.020
i. moist mucous membranes

Possible Nursing Interventions

- Keep accurate record of intake and output.
- Assess and record

   —IV fluids and condition of IV site every hour
   —signs/symptoms of fluid volume deficit (such as those listed under "Characteristics") every 2 hours and PRN
   —CVP every 1 or 2 hours and PRN
   —heart rate and blood pressure every hour and PRN

- Ensure that colloids are administered as ordered. Assess and record effectiveness.
- Check and record urine specific gravity every void or as ordered.
- If Foley catheter is in place, record hourly output. Maintain aseptic technique when emptying urine and administering catheter care.

Evaluation for Charting

- State intake and output.
- Describe condition of IV site.
- State highest and lowest heart rates and B/P and CVP values.

- Describe any signs/symptoms of fluid volume deficit (such as those listed under "Characteristics").
- Describe any therapeutic measures used to maintain adequate fluid volume and their effectiveness.
- State highest and lowest urine specific gravity values.

Nursing Diagnosis **IMPAIRED GAS EXCHANGE**

Definition Alteration in the exchange of oxygen and carbon dioxide in the lungs and/or at the cellular level

Possibly Related to

- Ineffective airway clearance secondary to edema and mechanical obstruction
- Damaged pulmonary tissue
- Increased pulmonary secretions secondary to smoke inhalation
- Pulmonary edema or embolus
- Bacterial pneumonia
- Restricted chest expansion

Characteristics Tachypnea

Hoarseness/drooling/inability to clear secretions

Crackles, rhonchi, and wheezing

Stridor

Dyspnea

Hypoxia

Cyanosis

Abnormal blood gas values

Retractions

Carbonaceous (black) sputum

Expected Outcomes Child will maintain adequate gas exchange as evidenced by

a. respiratory rate within acceptable range (state specific highest and lowest rate for each child)
b. ability to clear secretions

c. clear to white secretions
d. clear and equal breath sounds
e. lack of

—dyspnea
—cyanosis
—retractions

f. arterial pH of 7.35 to 7.45
g. PaCO2 of 35 to 45 mm Hg
h. PaO2 of 75 to 100 mm Hg

**Possible Nursing
Interventions**

- Assess and record the following every 1 to 2 hours and PRN

—respiratory rate
—breath sounds
—color
—signs/symptoms of impaired gas exchange (such as those listed under "Characteristics")

- Suction using sterile technique every 2 hours and PRN. Record amount and characteristics of secretions.
- Administer humidified oxygen in the correct amount and by the correct route. Assess and record effectiveness of therapy.
- Assess and record arterial blood gas values as ordered. Notify physician of any abnormalities.
- Ensure that bronchodilators (such as isoproterenol or terbutaline) and mucolytic agents (such as Mucomyst) are administered on schedule. Assess and record effectiveness and side effects (such as tachycardia and bronchospasm).
- Ensure that chest physiotherapy is being done effectively and on schedule. Record effectiveness.

- Assist child with coughing and deep breathing, i.e., use of bedside spirometer, when indicated.
- Elevate head of bed at a 30° angle.
- If child in intubated, check ventilator settings (FiO2, Rate, PIP or TV, PEEP/CPAP) every 15 minutes. Record every 1 to 2 hours.

Evaluation for Charting

- State highest and lowest respiratory rates.
- Describe breath sounds.
- Describe any signs/symptoms of impaired gas exchange (such as those listed under "Characteristics").
- State highest and lowest arterial blood gas values and state the ongoing physiological process (i.e., respiratory acidosis)
- State amount and route of oxygen delivery. Describe effectiveness.
- State frequency of suctioning and describe amount and characteristics of secretions.
- State whether chest physiotherapy was done on schedule. Describe child's response to chest physiotherapy and its effectiveness in improving gas exchange.
- State whether bronchodilators and mucolytic agents were administered on schedule. Describe effectiveness and any side effects.
- State whether head of bed was elevated.
- Describe any therapeutic measures used to improve gas exchange and their effectiveness.
- State type of endotracheal tube used and ventilator settings.

Nursing Diagnosis	**ALTERATION IN COMFORT**
Definition	A condition in which an individual experiences discomfort
Possibly Related to	• Thermal injury • Procedures/treatments

Characteristics	Constant crying
	Facial grimacing
	Physical signs/symptoms
	  Tachycardia
	  Tachypnea/bradypnea
	  Increased blood pressure
	Verbal communication of discomfort

Expected Outcomes	Child will be free of severe/constant discomfort as evidenced by

a. lack of constant crying
b. lack of facial expression of discomfort
c. heart rate within acceptable range (state specific highest and lowest rates for each child)
d. respiratory rate within acceptable range (state specific highest and lowest rates for each child)
e. blood pressure within acceptable range (state specific highest and lowest pressures for each child)
f. verbal communication of comfort

Possible Nursing Interventions

• Assess and record any signs/symptoms of discomfort (such as those listed under "Characteristics") every 2 to 4 hours.
• Handle child gently.
• Ensure that analgesics are administered on schedule. Assess and record effectiveness. Premedicate child before treatments as indicated.

- Encourage family members to stay and comfort child when possible.
- Allow family members to participate in the care of the child when possible.
- Use distraction measures (listening to radio) when appropriate.

Evaluation for Charting

- Describe any signs/symptoms of discomfort.
- State range of vital signs.
- Describe any successful measures used to reduce discomfort.
- Describe effectiveness of analgesics.

Related Nursing Diagnoses

POTENTIAL FOR INFECTION related to

a. impaired skin integrity
b. decreased resistance

ELECTROLYTE IMBALANCE related to

a. tissue damage secondary to burn injury
b. cellular losses

FEAR (CHILD'S) related to

a. treatments/procedures
b. hospitalization
c. accidental nature of injury
d. separation and isolation from family

POISONING

Pathophysiology

Poisoning is a common cause of death in children. Accidental poisonings occur most frequently in children under the age of five and usually involve the ingestion of medications or household chemicals. The deliberate overingestion of one or more substances occurs most commonly in adolescents, either during experimentation or as a suicidal gesture.

Acetaminophen poisoning is currently the most common type of poisoning in children. Other poisonous substances that are often ingested include plants, soap, detergents, vitamins, pesticides, lead, aspirin, and prescription medications such as barbiturates, opiates, and tricyclic antidepressants.

Hospitalization of a child who has ingested a poison is necessary to observe for signs and/or complications of poisoning and for laboratory evaluation. The body systems affected depend on the agent ingested. The child's vital functions must be maintained, and supportive care is essential for optimal recovery.

ACETAMINOPHEN

Primary Nursing Diagnosis

ALTERATION IN METABOLIC FUNCTION

Definition

Imbalance in the body of the utilization of specific biochemicals

Possibly Related to

Hepatic damage secondary to overdose

Characteristics   Nausea/vomiting
Anorexia
Diaphoresis
Pallor
Pain in upper right quadrant
Jaundice
Confusion
Stupor
Prolonged prothrombin time
Elevated SGOT, SGPT, bilirubin
Elevated serum acetaminophen level

**Expected
Outcomes**   Child will have adequate metabolic
function as evidenced by

    a. lack of signs/symptoms of altered
       metabolic function (such as those
       listed under "Characteristics")
    b. prothrombin time within accept-
       able range of 12 to 14 seconds
    c. SGOT within acceptable range of
       10 to 40 IU/liter
    d. SGPT within acceptable range of
       5 to 35 IU/liter
    e. total serum bilirubin of 0.2 to 1.0
       mg/dl
    f. serum acetaminophen level below
       150 µg/ml

**Possible Nursing
Interventions**   • Assess and record every 1 to 2 hours
      and PRN

      —level of consciousness
      —signs/symptoms of metabolic dys-
        function (such as those listed
        under "Characteristics")

    • Assess and record laboratory values
      as indicated. Notify physician of any
      abnormalities.
    • Keep accurate record of intake and
      output.

- Assess and record IV fluids and condition of IV site every hour.
- Initial treatment includes administration of ipecac and fluids to induce emesis. Administer only if child is alert and awake. If gastric lavage is indicated, use a large-bore tube.
- When the antidote (N-acetylcysteine/Mucomyst) is indicated, administer via nasogastric tube or by mouth (disguise taste if possible). If vomiting occurs within one hour after administration, repeat the dose. Assess and record effectiveness and any side effects (such as nausea and vomiting).

Evaluation for Charting

- Describe level of consciousness.
- Describe any signs/symptoms of metabolic dysfunction (such as those listed under "Characteristics").
- State highest and lowest laboratory values.
- State intake and output.
- Describe condition of IV site.
- Describe the effectiveness of any therapeutic measures used to correct metabolic dysfunction.

SALICYLATE

Primary Nursing Diagnosis

IMPAIRED GAS EXCHANGE

Definition

Alteration in the exchane of oxygen and carbon dioxide in the lungs and/or at the cellular level

Possibly Related to

Increase in the depth and rate of respirations resulting from the effect of the drug on the respiratory center

Characteristics

Hyperventilation
Respiratory alkalosis

Hyperpyrexia
Diaphoresis
Vomiting
Diarrhea
Confusion
Lethargy
Coma

Expected Outcomes

Child will have adequate gas exchange as evidenced by

a. clear and equal breath sounds
b. respiratory rate within acceptable range (state specific highest and lowest rates for each child)
c. arterial pH of 7.35 to 7.45
d. PaCO2 between 35 and 45 mm Hg
e. PaO2 between 75 and 100 mm Hg
f. arterial bicarbonate level between 22 and 28 mEq/liter
g. lack of signs/symptoms of impaired gas exchange (such as those listed under "Characteristics")
h. temperature between 36.5° and 37.2° C

Possible Nursing Interventions

• Assess and record the following every 1 to 2 hours and PRN

—respiratory rate and temperature
—signs/symptoms of impaired gas exchange (such as those listed under "Characteristics")

• Assess and record arterial blood gas values as ordered. Notify physician of any abnormalities.
• Administer humidified oxygen in the correct amount and route. Assess and record effectiveness of therapy.
• Elevate head of bed at a 30° angle.

Evaluation for Charting

- State highest and lowest respiratory rates and temperatures.
- Describe any signs/symptoms of impaired gas exchange (such as those listed under "Characteristics").
- State highest and lowest arterial blood gas values and state the ongoing physiologic process (i.e., respiratory alkalosis).
- State amount and route of oxygen delivery. Describe effectiveness.
- State whether head of bed was elevated.

Related Nursing Diagnoses

ALTERATION IN LEVEL OF CONSCIOUSNESS related to

    a. hepatic encephalopathy
    b. impaired gas exchange

DECREASED CARDIAC OUTPUT related to

    a. fluid volume deficit
    b. dysrhythmias
    c. bleeding tendencies secondary to prolonged prothrombin time

INEFFECTIVE FAMILY COPING related to

    a. accidental illness of child
    b. fear of child not recovering from ingestion
    c. guilt from the circumstances of the child's illness
    d. suicide attempt

KNOWLEDGE DEFICIT, PARENTAL, related to prevention and safety

SHOCK

Pathophysiology

Shock occurs when the body's circulatory homeostatic mechanism is disrupted and the body attempts to compensate for the resultant circulatory failure. Shock is a clinical syndrome characterized by impaired tissue perfusion, which leads to cellular metabolic dysfunction. Cellular oxygenation becomes inadequate and/or inadequate cellular utilization of oxygen occurs. Metabolic acidosis results as anaerobic glycosis is initiated, leading to an excess of lactic and pyruvic acids. Unless the hemodynamic and metabolic deterioration can be stopped, the child's condition may decline rapidly and death may ensue.

Each child in shock presents his/her own unique clinical picture. Three common pathophysiological processes can emerge during shock: 1) hypovolemia, 2) alterations in peripheral circulation, and 3) central or cardiogenic failure.

Hypovolemia may be actual or relative. Actual hypovolemia results from situations leading to: 1) blood loss, as in trauma or gastrointestinal and intracranial hemorrhage, 2) plasma loss, as in burns or peritonitis, and 3) water loss, as in gastroenteritis or glycosuric diuresis. Relative hypovolemia results from an acute loss of peripheral vascular resistance. In hypovolemia, the reduction in blood/fluid volume causes a decreased venous return, low central venous pressure, reduced stroke volume, low cardiac output, a fall in blood pressure, and tachycardia.

The body responds to these changes by putting several compensatory mechanisms into action. The compensatory mechanisms attempt to conserve fluid and support the decreasing blood volume and blood pressure by increasing peripheral vascular resistance and shunting blood from the periphery to the heart and brain.

Changes in the peripheral circulation can secondarily contribute to alterations in the hemodynamic homeostatis of the shock patient. DIC, pooling of blood in the periphery, and abnormal permeability of the capillaries are all circulatory changes that can lead to the loss of plasma water and blood volume. The patient with sepsis, endotoxinemia, or trauma unassociated with hemorrhage can demonstrate these changes in the peripheral circulation.

In children, circulatory failure caused by cardiac failure is the least common. Cardiac failure can result from congenital heart disease, intracardiac shunting, inflow or outflow obstructions, or dysrhythmias.

The goal of treatment for the child in shock is to prevent/correct hypoperfusion and hypoxia and to preserve the function of all organs. The earlier that shock is diagnosed and treatment is initiated, the better the child's prognosis.

ALTERATION IN TISSUE PERFUSION: PERIPHERAL, CARDIOPULMONARY, CEREBRAL, RENAL

Primary Nursing Diagnosis

Definition Inadequate amount of blood and oxygen being delivered to the tissues in the body

Possibly Related to	Circulatory failure secondary to

- hypovolemia
- alterations in peripheral circulation
- cardiac failure

Characteristics   *Peripheral*
Cool, pale, clammy skin
Dry, pale mucous membranes
Diaphoresis
Poor skin turgor
Prolonged capillary refill
Cardiopulmonary
Tachycardia
Irregular heart rate
Thready, weak pulse
Decreased systolic blood pressure
Increased diastolic blood pressure
Hypotension
Narrowing pulse pressure
Decreased CVP
Tachypnea
Grey color
Cerebral
Restlessness
Confusion
Lethargy
Nausea
Thirst
Coma
Renal
Decreased urinary output

Expected Outcomes   Child will have adequate tissue perfusion as evidenced by
Peripheral

a. skin warm to touch
b. moist mucous membranes
c. rapid skin recoil

d. brisk capillary refill, within 2 to 3 seconds
e. lack of diaphoresis and pallor

Cardiopulmonary

a. heart rate within acceptable range (state specific highest and lowest rates for each child)
b. normal sinus rhythm
c. blood pressure within acceptable range (state specific highest and lowest pressures for each child)
d. pulse pressure within acceptable limits of 20 to 50 mm Hg
e. CVP within acceptable range of 4 to 8 mm Hg
f. respiratory rate within acceptable range (state specific highest and lowest rates for each child)
g. strong and equal peripheral pulses
h. lack of greyness

Cerebral

a. alertness when awake
b. orientation ×3 (if age-appropriate)
c. lack of

—extreme restlessness
—nausea
—excessive thirst

RENAL

a. adequate urine output (state specific highest and lowest output for each child; normal, 1 to 2 ml/kg/hour

Possible Nursing Interventions

• Assess and record every 1 to 2 hours and PRN

—vital signs
—CVP

—color

—level of consciousness

—signs/symptoms of alteration in tissue perfusion (such as those listed under "Characteristics")

- Keep accurate record of intake and output. If Foley Catheter is in place, keep hourly output. Maintain aseptic technique when emptying urine and administering catheter care.
- Evaluate and record results of EKG strips at least once/shift.
- Administer oxygen in the correct amount and route. Assess and record effectiveness of therapy.
- Ensure that volume expanders, fluids, and blood products are administered as ordered (such as albumin, Ringer's lactate, and packed red blood cells), depending on the type of shock. Assess and record effectiveness.
- Ensure that medications are administered as ordered (such as antibiotics, sympathomimetics, vasodilators, and inotropic agents), depending on the type of shock. Assess and record effectiveness and any side effects.

Evaluation for Charting

- Describe any signs/symptoms of altered tissue perfusion (such as those listed under "Characteristics").
- State range of vital signs, including CVP.
- Describe the child's color.
- State intake and output.
- Document EKG interpretation.
- State amount and route of oxygen delivery. Describe effectiveness.

- Describe any therapeutic measures used to improve tissue perfusion and their effectiveness.

Nursing Diagnosis	**IMPAIRED GAS EXCHANGE**
Definition	Alteration in the exchange of oxygen and carbon dioxide in the lungs and/or at the cellular level
Possibly Related to	Tissue hypoxia secondary to circulatory failure
Characteristics	Hypoxemia
	Hypercapnia
	Respiratory acidosis
	Tachypnea
	Dyspnea
	Pallor/Grey color
	Cyanosis

Expected Outcomes

Child will maintain adequate gas exchange as evidenced by

a. PaO_2 between 75 and 100 mm Hg
b. $PaCO_2$ between 20 and 25 mm Hg
c. arterial pH between 7.35 and 7.45
d. respiratory rate within acceptable range (state specific highest and lowest rates for each child)
e. lack of

—dyspnea
—pallor/grey color
—cyanosis

Possible Nursing Interventions

- Assess and record arterial blood gas values as ordered. Notify physician of any abnormalities.
- Assess and record every 1 to 2 hours and PRN

—respiratory rate

—signs/symptoms of impaired gas exchange (such as those listed under "Characteristics")

—color

- Administer humidified oxygen in the correct amount and by the correct route. Asssess and record effectiveness of therapy.
- If child is intubated, check ventilator settings (FiO2, Rate, PIP or RV, PEEP/CPAP) every 15 minutes. Record every 1 to 2 hours. Suction using sterile technique every 2 hours and PRN. Record amount and characteristics of secretions.
- Elevate head of bed at a 30° angle.

Evaluation for Charting

- State highest and lowest arterial blood gas values and state the ongoing physiological process (i.e., respiratory acidosis).
- State highest and lowest respiratory rates.
- Describe any signs/symptoms of impaired gas exchange (such as those listed under "Characteristics").
- State amount and route of oxygen delivery. Describe effectiveness.
- State type of endotracheal tube used and ventilator settings.
- State frequency of suctioning and describe amount and characteristics of secretions.
- State whether head of bed was elevated.
- Describe any therapeutic measures used to improve gas exchange and their effectiveness.

Related Nursing Diagnoses

FLUID VOLUME DEFICIT related to hypovolemia

ELECTROLYTE IMBALANCE related to

a. hypovolemia
b. tissue damage

ALTERATION IN NUTRITION: LESS THAN BODY REQUIREMENTS related to impaired tissue perfusion

INEFFECTIVE FAMILY COPING related to

a. severity of illness
b. unknown prognosis

Medical Diagnosis	# SUDDEN INFANT DEATH SYNDROME (SIDS), NEAR-MISS
Pathophysiology	Sudden infant death syndrome (SIDS) is the leading cause of nonaccidental death in infants between the ages of one week and one year. It usually occurs before six months of age and during the infant's sleep. In the United States, SIDS claims the life of approximately two in every 1000 births. The diagnosis of SIDS is made when an infant dies unexpectedly, the death is not explainable by the medical history, and no adequate cause of death is found in a postmortem examination.
	The cause of SIDS remains unknown. There do seem to be several physiologic factors, such as alterations in the control mechanisms of sleep, respiration, and cardiac rhythm, that have led to the formation of numerous theories.
	"Near-miss" infants are SIDS victims who have been successfully resuscitated.
Primary Nursing Diagnosis	## INEFFECTIVE BREATHING PATTERN
Definition	A breathing pattern that results in oxygen insufficient to meet the cellular requirements of the body
Possibly Related to Characteristics	Unknown cause Apnea Cyanosis Hypoxia Pallor Cold, clammy skin Flaccidity

**Expected
Outcomes**   Child will have an effective breathing
pattern as evidenced by

    a. respiratory rate within acceptable
    range (state specific highest and
    lowest rate for each child)
    b. lack of

    —cyanosis
    —pallor
    —flaccidity

    c. skin warm and dry to touch

**Possible Nursing
Interventions** • Assess and record every 2 hours and
PRN

    —respiratory rate
    —infant's color
    —infant's muscle tone
    —temperature and dryness of skin

• Ensure that sleeping infant remains
on apnea monitor with alarms appropriately set. Record the frequency,
duration, and type of stimulation
needed for any apneic episodes.
• Assist with pneumogram as indicated.
• Ensure that medications (such as
terbutaline) are administered on
schedule if ordered. Assess and record effectiveness and any side effects (such as tachycardia).
• If infant is intubated

    —check ventilator settings (FiO2,
    Rate, PIP or TV, PEEP/CPAP) ev-
    ery 15 minutes. Record every 1 to
    2 hours.
    —suction using sterile technique
    PRN

- State highest and lowest respiratory rate.
- Describe infant's color, muscle tone, and temperature and dryness of skin.
- Describe any apneic episodes and type and effectiveness of stimulation.
- State whether medications were given on schedule. Describe effectiveness and any side effects.
- State type of endotracheal tube used and ventilator settings.
- State frequency of suctioning and describe characteristics.

Nursing Diagnosis

INEFFECTIVE FAMILY COPING

Definition

Inability of family members to manage problems and concerns effectively

Possibly Related to

- Unexpectedness of illness
- Unknown cause of illness
- Possible sequelae
- Hospitalization in intensive care unit
- Guilt (unfounded)

Characteristics

Inability to leave the infant

Inappropriate anger toward staff members

Inappropriate anger toward other family members or significant others (i.e., babysitter)

Inability to meet own basic needs such as eating and resting

Inability to express fears and concerns

Inability to ask for and accept outside help

Failure to understand repeated explanations regarding the illness, treatments, and procedures

Expected Outcomes

Family will be able to cope appropriately as evidenced by

a. being able to leave the infant for short periods especially to care for own basic needs such as eating meals and getting rest

b. expressing anger appropriately toward staff or others, verbalization that initial anger had been inappropriate

c. being able to express fears and concerns to members of the health care team

d. knowing when it is appropriate to accept outside help

e. verbalizing understanding of explanations regarding the illness, treatments, and procedures

Possible Nursing Interventions

- Communicate with family concerning their infant's condition at least once/shift and PRN as the infant's condition demands. This may require telephoning the family when they are not able to come to the hospital.

- Encourage family to express their feelings, fears, and concerns.

- Assist and encourage family to meet own basic needs, such as eating and resting appropriately.

- Identify and record any past or usually successful coping strategies used by the family.

- Provide the family with outside help or assist them in seeking outside help when indicated.

- Explain the course of the illness, treatments, and procedures to the family. Include reasons for treatments and procedures.

**Evaluation
for Charting**

- State whether family members were able to leave the infant long enough to meet their own basic needs.
- Describe any feelings, fears, and concerns expressed by the family.
- State whether the family is willing to accept outside help as indicated.
- State whether the family was able to understand the infant's illness to the best of their ability.
- State whether the family was able to understand the necessity and rationale for treatments and procedures.
- State any successful measures used to help family's coping ability.

**Related Nursing
Diagnoses**

ALTERATION IN LEVEL OF CONSCIOUSNESS related to hypoxia secondary to apnea

DECREASED CARDIAC OUTPUT related to

a. apnea
b. dysrhythmias

GROWTH AND DEVELOPMENTAL DELAY related to brain damage secondary to anoxic episodes

GRIEVING, ANTICIPATORY related to the possiblity of death

Section 3
Additional Nursing Diagnoses

Nursing Diagnosis	# ACTIVITY INTOLERANCE
Definition	Insufficient psychosocial, emotional, or physiologic ability to perform required or desired activities
Possibly Related to	Fatigue, weakness secondary to

- disease process
- compromised oxygen transport
- electrolyte imbalance
- circulatory compromise
- status/post-surgical procedure
- pain
- depression
- lack of motivation

Characteristics

Verbalization of weakness or fatigue

Decreased endurance

Decreased muscle tone

Impaired ability to perform activities of daily living

Impaired ability to ambulate or reposition self

Dyspnea

Shortness of breath

Increased, weak pulse

Expected Outcomes

Infant/child will have appropriate activity tolerance for age as evidenced by

a. age-appropriate activity endurance
b. appropriate strength of muscle tone
c. ability to perform activities of daily living
d. ability to ambulate and reposition self
e. strong heart rate within acceptable range (state specific highest and lowest rate for each infant/child)

Possible Nursing Interventions

f. lack of
   —verbalization of weakness or fatigue
   —dyspnea
   —shortness of breath

- Organize care to provide rest periods.
- Assist with activities of daily living, ambulation, and repositioning.
- Assess and record baseline and activity vital signs every 4 hours and PRN.
- Assist infant/child with slowly increasing activity level when indicated.
- Ensure that infant/child is receiving and tolerating adequate nutritional support.
- Ensure that vitamins are administered on schedule if ordered.
- Perform passive range of motion when indicated. Record infant/child's tolerance of procedure.

Evaluation for Charting

- State whether infant/child was able to have uninterrupted rest periods throughout the shift.
- Describe infant/child's ability to participate in activities of daily living, ambulation, and repositioning.
- State range of baseline and activity vital signs.
- Describe infant/child's nutritional intake and tolerance.
- State whether vitamins were administered on schedule.
- Describe infant/child's tolerance of range of motion procedure.

Nursing Diagnosis	# ANTICIPATORY GRIEVING: PARENTAL/FAMILY
Definition	Feelings of deep sadness and distress
Possibly Related to	• Critical state of infant/child illness • Separation from infant/child • Physical defect of infant/child • Developmental or cognitive impairment of infant/child • Infant/child death
Characteristics	Verbal expression of grief by parents/ family Sadness Crying, screaming Inability to carry on with activities of daily living at an optimal level Need for repeated explanations and reassurance Passivity
Expected Outcomes	Parents/family will grieve appropriately as evidenced by

      a. crying quietly
      b. talking and asking questions about the infant/child
      c. seeking help and advice appropriately
      d. performing activities of daily living at an optimal level

Possible Nursing Interventions

- Allow parents/family to grieve in their own way and give them support.
- Encourage parents/family to spend time with their infant/child if it seems to help their grieving process.
- If possible, have the same nurse(s) care for infant/child from day to day

to provide consistent feedback for family.

- Allow parents/family to participate in the care of the infant/child when possible (dressing changes, bath, baptism, changing diapers, feeding, etc.).
- Allow parents/family to spend time alone at their infant/child's bedside if possible.
- Spend time with the parents/family when possible.
- Keep parents/family up to date on the condition of their infant.
- When possible, have family make tapes of their voices that can be played for infant/child.
- Allow parents/family to photograph their infant/child when appropriate.

Evaluation for Charting
- State whether parents/family verbalized any feelings of grief.
- Describe any signs/symptoms of grief displayed by parents/family (such as those listed under "Characteristics").
- State whether parents/family were able to carry on with activities of daily living.
- Describe any successful measures used to help parents/family cope with their grief.

Primary Nursing Diagnosis	# DEVELOPMENTAL DELAY
Definition	Failure to progress in expected tasks and skills according to chronologic age
Possibly Related to	• Increased intracranial pressure • Cerebrovascular infarcts • Metabolic disorders • Environmental problems (e.g., lack of stimulation) • Nutritional deficit • Parental knowledge deficit • Repeated or long-term hospitalization • Chronic or terminal illness

Characteristics	Will vary with age and state of development of each child (refer to a growth and development chart); for example, a 3-month-old infant would
	    Hold head up when placed on abdomen
	    Follow objects
	    Regard face of others
	    Smile responsively
	    Manifest Moro, sucking, and rooting reflexes

Expected Outcomes	Child will progress developmentally as evidenced by
	  a. lack of markedly regressed behavior
	  b. continuation of preillness activities
	  c. attainment of developmental milestones according to age
	
	Parents will describe specific tasks/skills that child is able to do.

Possible Nursing Interventions	• Allow child to move around in bed/crib when possible.

- If restraints are needed, remove restraints when child can be monitored constantly.
- Put familiar washable articles, such as toys and favorite blanket, in the bed/crib with the child.
- Provide age-appropriate activities and/or stimulation for child, such as mobile, television, music box, or radio.
- Use play therapy when appropriate.
- If possible, allow child to participate in activities of daily living.
- For children who are school-aged, assist in arranging for child to continue with school work when possible.
- Assist family in helping child to progress developmentally by suggesting developmentally appropriate activities and toys.
- Encourage family to continue setting some limits on child's behavior while hospitalized so the child will feel secure.

Evaluation for Charting

- Describe any developmental delays or regressed behavior.
- Describe child's level of developmental tasks/skills attainment.
- Describe any successful measures used to help child attain developmental milestones.

Nursing Diagnosis	# IMPAIRED VERBAL COMMUNICATION
Definition	Inability of individual to use or understand verbal messages
Possibly Related to	• Anatomical defect (cleft lip/palate) • Cerebral impairment • Nervous system disorder • Physical obstruction (endotracheal tube, tracheostomy, tumor) • Cultural difference
Characteristics	Weak or absent voice Inability to speak same language Articulation problems
Expected Outcomes	Infant/child will be able to communicate verbally as evidenced by a. audible voice b. ability to speak and understand same language c. lack of articulation problems
Possible Nursing Interventions	• Assess and record infant/child's ability to communicate verbally every shift and PRN. Observe and record nonverbal cues. • Anticipate infant/child's needs when possible. • Ask yes or no questions when appropriate. • Provide alternative forms of communication (i.e., alphabet board, paper and pencil, flash cards, eye blinking, etc.). • Record effectiveness of any alternative method used. • Provide positive feedback for attempts at communication.

Evaluation for Charting

- Describe infant/child's ability to communicate.
- Describe any nonverbal cues used by infant/child.
- Describe any therapeutic measures used and their effectiveness in improving communication.

IMPAIRMENT OF SKIN INTEGRITY

Definition Interruption in integrity of the skin

Possibly Related to

- Fragile tissue
- Decreased amount of brown fat
- Dehydration
- Edema
- Infections
- Alteration in metabolic function
- Impaired gas exchange
- Impaired circulation
- Thermal injury
- Decreased tissue perfusion

Characteristics Discoloration of skin (reddened area)
Open or draining areas on skin
Change in elasticity of skin
Lesions
Pruritus

Expected Outcomes Infant/child will be free of signs/symptoms of impaired skin integrity as evidenced by

a. natural skin color
b. clean, intact skin
c. lack of

—reddened areas or discoloration
—open or draining areas
—change in elasticity
—lesions
—pruritis

Possible Nursing Interventions

- Handle infant/child gently.
- Encourage others (e.g., parents, visitors, x-ray personnel) to handle infant/child gently.
- Bathe daily (or as indicated) with water. Use soap when indicated.

- Use lotion to moisturize skin when indicated. Lotion is contraindicated if infant is under infant warmer.
- Decrease use of tape and electrodes when possible.
- Carefully remove tape and electrodes when necessary. Use adhesive tape remover when available.
- Assess and record skin condition every shift. Report any abnormalities to the physician.
- Reposition infant/child every 2 hours unless contraindicated.
- Consider using sheepskin blankets, water beds, egg crates, etc.
- Change diaper/linens as soon as possible after elimination or soiling.
- Treat any existing or potential breakdown/wound areas as soon as they are discovered by keeping area clean and dry, exposing area to air if indicated, and applying medication or ointment, if ordered.

Evaluation for Charting

- Describe any potential or actual areas of skin breakdown.
- Describe any therapeutic measures used to prevent or correct impaired skin integrity.

Bibliography

Avery, M. E., & Frantz, I. D., III (1983). To breathe or not to breathe. What have we learned about apneic spells and sudden infant death? *The New England Journal of Medicine, 309* (2), 107–108.

Axton, S. E. (1986). *Neonatal and pediatric care plans.* Baltimore: Williams & Wilkins.

Barnett, D. J. (1988). The clinician's guide to pediatric AIDS. *Contemporary Pediatrics, 5,* 24–47.

Barrett, E. J., & DeFranzo, R. A. (1984, April). Diabetic ketoacidosis: Diagnosis and treatment. *Hospital Practice, 19* (4), 89–104.

Blanchet, E. D. (Ed.). (1988). *AIDS: A health care management response.* Rockville, MD: Aspen.

Boland, M., & Gaskill, T. D. B. (1984). Managing AIDS in children. *The American Journal of Maternal/Child Nursing, 9,* 384–389.

Calcagno, P. L., Subramanian, S., & Sostek, A. M. (1984). Sudden infant death syndrome. *University Case Studies, 1* (1).

Calcagno, P. L., Subramanian, S., & Sostek, A. M. (1984). Sudden infant death syndrome. *University Case Studies, 1* (2).

Carpenito, L. J. (1987). *Handbook of nursing diagnosis* (2nd ed.). Philadelphia: Lippincott.

Cooke, S. S. (1986). Major thermal injury—the first 48 hours. *Critical Care Nurse, 6* (1), 55–63.

Cowan, M. J., Hellman, D., Chudwin, D., Wara, D. W., Chang, R. S., & Ammann, A. J. (1984). Maternal transmission of acquired immune deficiency syndrome. *Pediatrics, 73* (3), 382–386.

Cunningham, M. (1987). Intraventricular hemorrhage in the premature. *Dimensions of Critical Care Nursing, 6* (1), 20–27.

Drummond, K. N. (1985). Hemolytic uremic syndrome—then and now. *The New England Journal of Medicine, 312* (2), 116–118.

Durham, J. D., & Cohen, F. L. (Eds.). (1987). *The person with AIDS: Nursing perspectives.* New York: Springer.

Fink, B. W. (1975). *Congenital heart disease.* Chicago: Year Book Publishers.

Fischback, F. T. (1984). *A manual of laboratory diagnostic tests* (2nd ed.). Philadelphia: Lippincott.

Fochhtman, D., & Raffensperger, J. G. (1976). *Principles of nursing care for the pediatric surgery patient* (2nd ed.). Boston: Little, Brown.

Foster, D. W., & McGarry, J. D. (1983). The metabolic derangements and treatment of diabetic ketoacidosis. *The New England Journal of Medicine, 309* (3), 159–168.

Frumkin, L. R., & Leonard, J. M. (1987). *Questions and answers on AIDS*. Oradell, NJ: Medical Economics Books.

Goldstein, B., & Todres, I. D. (Eds.). (1987). *Massachusetts General Hospital Pediatric Intensive Care Unit Housestaff Manual*.

Gordon, M. (1985). *Manual of nursing diagnosis, 1984–1985*. New York: McGraw-Hill.

Graves, S. A. (1984). Near drowning. *Pediatric Emergency Casebook, 3* (1).

Gregory, S. E. B. (1987), April). Air leak syndromes. *Neonatal Network*, 40–46.

Grippi, C., Ward, L., & Roncoli, M. (1988, May). The case of baby Alice: AIDS/ARC in infancy. *Neonatal Network*, 9–14.

Hazinski, M. F. (1984). *Nursing care of the critically ill child*. St. Louis: Mosby.

Heiss, R. (1987). Immunology of AIDS. *Pediatric Annals, 16* (6), 495–503.

Ingersoll, G. L., & Leyden, D. B. (1987). The Glasgow Coma Scale for patients with head injuries. *Critical Care Nurse, 7* (5), 26–32.

Inglis, A. D., & Lozano, M. (1986). AIDS and the neonatal ICU. *Neonatal Network, 5* (3), 39–43.

James, S. R., & Mott, S. R. (1988). *Child health nursing*. Reading, MA: Addison-Wesley.

Johnson, B. C., Wells, S. J., Hoffmeister, D., & Dungca, C. U. (1988). *Standards for critical care* (3rd ed.). St. Louis: Mosby.

Kelly, D. H. (1983). SIDS and Near-SIDS. *Pediatric Emergency Casebook, 1* (5).

Kim, M. J., McFarland, G. K., & McLane, A. M. (1987). *Pocket guide to nursing diagnoses*. St. Louis: Mosby.

Klaus, M. H., & Franaroff, A. A. (1979). *Care of the high-risk neonate* (2nd ed.). Philadelphia: Saunders.

Korones, S. B. (1981). *High-risk newborn infant: The basis of intensive nursing care* (3rd ed.). St. Louis: Mosby.

Kreisberg, R. A. (1978). Diabetic ketoacidosis: New concepts and trends in pathogenesis and treatment. *Annals of Internal Medicine, 88,* 681–695.

Leahey, M., & Wright, L. M. (1987). *Families and life-threatening illness.* Springhouse, PA: Springhouse.

LeBoeuf, M. B., & Greco-Gallagher, M. (1987). Standardized care plan for the child with bacterial meningitis. *Critical Care Nurse, 7* (5), 66–76.

Levine, M. I., & Heavenrich, R. M. (Eds.). (1984). Sudden infant death syndrome and infantile apnea: Medical and psychosocial aspects of management. *Pediatric Annals, 13,* 3.

Malsteed, R. T. (1985). *Pharmacology: Drug therapy and nursing considerations* (2nd ed.). Philadelphia: Lippincott.

Manginello, F. P. (1986). Necrotizing enterocolitis. *Pediatric Emergency Casebook, 4* (2).

Metheny, N. M. (1987). *Fluid and electrolyte balance: Nursing considerations.* Philadelphia: Lippincott.

Moses, A. M. (1977, July). Diabetes insipidus and ADH regulation. *Hospital Practice,* 37–44.

Muscari, M. E. (1987). Adolescent suicide attempts by acetaminophen ingestion. *The American Journal of Maternal/Child Nursing, 12,* 32–35.

Nelson, N. P., & Beckel, J. (Eds.). (1987). *Nursing care plans for the pediatric patient.* St. Louis: Mosby.

New nursing skillbook: Monitoring fluid and electrolytes precisely (2nd ed.). (1984). Springhouse, PA: Springhouse.

Oellrich, R. G. (1985). Pneumothorax, chest tubes, and the neonate. *The American journal of Maternal/Child Nursing, 10,* 29–35.

Orlowski, J. P. (Ed.). (1980). Symposium on pediatric intensive care. *The Pediatric Clinics of North America, 27* (3).

Orlowski, J. P. (Ed.). (1987). Intensive care. *The Pediatric Clinics of North America, 34* (1).

Pollack-Latham, C. L. (1987). Intracranial pressure monitoring: Part 1—Physiologic principles. *Critical Care Nurse, 7* (5), 40–52.

Robbins, S. L. (1984). *Pathologic basis of disease.* Philadelphia: Saunders.

Schartz, S. I., Shires, G. T., Spencer, F. C., & Storer, E. H. (1979). *Principles of surgery* (3rd ed.). New York: McGraw-Hill.

Smith, J. B. (Ed.). (1983). *Pediatric critical care.* New York: Wiley.

Smith-Blair, N., & Stephson, C. (1986). Gastoschisis, a nursing perspective. *Focus on Critical Care, 13* (2), 9–19.

Stahler-Miller, K. (1983). *Neonatal and pediatric critical care nursing.* New York: Chuchhill Livingstone.

Swearingen, P. L. (Ed.). (1986). *Manual of nursing therapeutics: Applying nursing diagnoses to medical disorders.* Menlo Park, CA: Addison-Wesley.

Synopsis of Pediatric Emergencies. (1986, November). Tenth Annual Pediatrics Postgraduate Conference. Texas Tech University Health Sciences Center, Lubbock, TX.

Thorn, G. W., Addams, R. D., Braunwald, E., Isselbacher, K. J., & Petersdorf, R. G. (1977). *Principles of internal medicine* (8th ed.). New York: McGraw-Hill.

Thurkauf, G. E. (1987). Acetaminophen overdose. *Critical Care Nurse, 7* (1), 20–29.

Vanden Belt, R. J., Ronan, J. A., & Bedynek, J. L. (1979). *Cardiology: A clinical approach.* Chicago: Year Book Medical Publishers.

Vestal, K. W., & McKenzie, C. A. M. (1983). *High-risk perinatal nursing.* Philadelphia: Saunders.

Vulcan, B. M. (1987). Acute bacterial meningitis in infancy and childhood. *Critical Care Nurse, 7* (5), 53–65.

Walsh, M. C., & Kliegman, R. M. (1986). Necrotizing enterocolitis: Treatment based on staging criteria. *Pediatric Clinics of North America, 33* (1), 179–201.

Whaley, L. F., & Wong, D. L. (1987). *Nursing care of infants and children* (3rd ed.). St. Louis: Mosby.

Zimmerman, S. S., & Gildea, J. H. (Eds.). (1985). *Critical care pediatrics.* Philadelphia: Saunders.

Index